I0042686

John Bell

Engravings explaining the anatomy of the bones, muscles and joints

John Bell

Engravings explaining the anatomy of the bones, muscles and joints

ISBN/EAN: 9783741103988

Manufactured in Europe, USA, Canada, Australia, Japa

Cover: Foto ©Lupo / pixelio.de

Manufactured and distributed by brebook publishing software
(www.brebook.com)

John Bell

Engravings explaining the anatomy of the bones, muscles and joints

ENGRAVINGS,

EXPLAINING THE

ANATOMY

OF THE

BONES, MUSCLES, AND JOINTS.

BY

JOHN BELL, Surgeon.

EDINBURGH:

PRINTED BY JOHN PATERSON;

FOR BELL AND BRADFUTE, AND T. DUNCAN; AND J. JOHNSON,
AND G. G. G. & J. ROBINSONS, LONDON.

MDCCXCIV.

In a Book containing fo many thoufand technical terms, it will not be particular though the Student fhould find more to correct than what is here put down.—But thefe are fome of the chief errata; and, fince many of them affect the fenfe, the Student fhould touch them with the pen before he begins to read.

ERRATA.

Page
4. *line* 7. *for* ftretches *read* unites it.
8. *line* 1. *for* lefs *read* leffer.
31. *line* 15. *for* 4 *read* 6.
35. *line* 13. *for* futures *read* future.
Ibid. line 13. *for* feparate *read* feparates.
Ibid. line 14. *for* Œthmoid *read* Clinoid.
54. *line* 20. *for* d. d. *read* æ. æ.
55. *line* 17. *for* Pubis *read* Ifchium.
69. *line* 22. *for* inner *read* outer.
72. *line* 7. *for* Radius *read* Humerus.
97 *line* 15. *for* cartilages *read* cartilage.
Ibid. lines 18, 19 *for* 44. 45. 46. *read* 54. 55. 56.
98. *line* 4. *for* ix. *read* x.
100. *line* 1. *for* Sterno-hyoideus *read* Sterno-thyroideus.
Ibid. line 22. *for* Arytenoideus obliquus *read* Arytenoideus lateralis
101. *line* 16, *for* Styloid mufcle *read* Styloid procefs.

Page
110. *lin. ult. for* uncovered by the fkin *read* uncovered of the fkin.
119. *line* 7. *dele* Below the fpine is feen the Infrafpinatus.
134. *line* 6. *for* where *read* whence.
146. *line* 14. for d. d. *read* b. b.
156. *line* 18. *for* iii. *read* iv.
159. *line* 2. *from foot, for* 188. *read* 186.
168. *line* 7. *for* Coraco brachialis *read* Biceps.
173. *line* 4. *for* wrift *read* creft.
174. *line* 7. *for* cancellæ *read* lamellæ.
175. *line* 6. for (g) *read* (9).
Ibid. line 21. for (s) *read* (m).
177. *line* 15. for (m) *read* (u).
190 *line* 2. *for* outer *read* inner.
Ibid. line 10. *dele* often.
191. *line* 4. *for* fubftained *read* fuftained.

TO

Dr. DANIEL RUTHERFORD,

PROFESSOR OF MEDICINE AND BOTANY,

AND

PHYSICIAN TO THE ROYAL INFIRMARY,

EDINBURGH.

SIR,

In prefenting this Book of Plates to one who is fo well able as you are to judge of their defects, I ought to add fome value to the offering, by declaring the motives of it.—It is a mark of gratitude for the friendly care with which, in company with my worthy Mafter, you watched over me during a long and dangerous illnefs. Perhaps there can be no higher compliment betwixt medical men, than this confidence in time of ficknefs; and furely, if I may judge from my own feelings, nothing can be more grateful than the remembrance of kindneffes beftowed at fuch a time.——May your fkill be long ufeful to your fellow-citizens; and may it be always valued as I value it.

I am,

SIR,

With refpect,

Your Friend, and Humble Servant,

JOHN BELL.

PREFACE.

WHEN a young man, who had been blind from his childifh
years, had his fight reftored to him by our celebrated furgeon CHESSELDEN, all his thoughts, and feelings, and pleafures,
and pains, were very interefting to his friends; for that moft delightful of all our fenfes was to him as a dream of fairy vifions,
confufed, yet delightful, beyond all that the fancy can conceive.
" He was like one newly born into the world, needing to learn
" anew all the objects around him, knowing nothing by the eye,
" but all by the touch. It was long before he found out that pic-
" tures reprefented folid bodies, and then he was much furprifed
" that thofe things, which to the eye feemed prominent and round,
" were to the touch quite even and flat; he afked his friends which
" was indeed the lying fenfe, feeling or feeing."

a   " Being

" Being fhown his father's picture in a locket, at his mother's
" watch, and told what it was, he acknowledged a likenefs, but
" was vaftly furprifed ; afking, how it could be that a large face
" could be expreffed in fo little room; faying, it fhould have feemed
" as impoffible to him, as to have put a bufhel of any thing into a
" pint."

Now there are many, who having enjoyed and ufed this precious
fenfe during all their lives, have never come to know, like this
young man, that, even within the narroweft circle, the reprefentation is as perfect and true, as in the full fize of the human body ;
foolifhly imagining that nothing can be drawn but of its natural
fize. If a man were to take this fancy, that nothing of anatomy
could be drawn but of the full fize of life, with what high contempt
muft he look down upon thefe little plates ; where I have endeavoured to reprefent, in this miniature form, what it muft be con-
feffed, might be more fully reprefented on a larger fcale: and yet
I am fenfible, that thofe, who cannot underftand thefe plates,
will hardly profit even by that ftately anatomical figure of full
fix feet high, which, being cut in copper, with googes, and chif-
fels, and mallets, and all kinds of inftruments, muft eftablifh a reputation for its author; which, if not high, will not fail to be
at leaft of a lafting kind ; neither apt to be forgotten, nor liable,
like other difcoveries, to go aftray.

2   As

" As I proceeded in writing a book of anatomy, I felt more
" and more, at every ftep, the neceffity of giving plates to it ;"
for a book of anatomy without thefe feemed to me no better than
a book of geography without its maps ; it was, in my mind, like
teaching mathematics without diagrams, or folving Euclid's pro-
blems without the help of figures or lines, by the mere force of
imagination alone.   Indeed any one, who, ftudying without fome
help of plates, tries to underftand and to remember an anatomical
defcription with no other reprefentation than words merely, will
feel, that he is like one attempting to work a rule of arithmetic
without the ufe of cyphers, trying to remember the value and
denomination of each part throughout the whole train of numbers ; he is ingenious in difficulties, making an abftract fubject
of one belonging to the fenfes chiefly, and attempting to obtain
by words, thofe ideas which muft come to him only through the eye.

It was while I was writing anatomical defcriptions that I firft
thought of drawings, and of placing my fubjects in thofe very
fhapes and poftures in which they were explained :—and I conceived, that the defcriptions and the drawings might thus be wrought
into one perfect whole; being as two parts of one idea, or as one idea
prefented in a double form, once to the eye, and once again to the ear.
If, in any material points, my drawings and defcriptions fhall thus
agree, then muft the ideas be made out to my reader clear and fair;
and fhould infinuate themfelves into his mind without labour or

thought

thought on his part; while he is not toiling from defcriptions to drawings; not harraffed with continual interruptions, incongruous ideas, parts defcribed but not reprefented, or reprefented and not defcribed; not travelling far and wide from the ideas of one author, to the reprefentation of another; never trying to affociate ideas which have no affinity, nor ftriving to bring drawings and defcriptions together which are as far, as may be, from being parts of the fame idea, or from being capable of that clofe comparifon which the ftudent feeks, and miffes with a difappointment which is continually renewed. Such muft be the ftudent's labour, (a labour which might well opprefs the moft active mind,) if the teacher be not careful to preferve for him this correfpondence of ideas; whether he be employed in comparing his lecture with the fubject lying before him, or his drawings with his book.

From the firft dawnings of anatomical knowledge, or at leaft from the very earlieft invention of anatomical plates, this vitious practice has prevailed, that each author, carelefs of this correfpondence of ideas; never thinking of the harmony that ought ftill to fubfift between thofe notions which are to be conveyed by words, and thofe which fpeak to the eye, in the truer language of this fubject; intending merely to write a book, and rather with the hopes of procuring himfelf a name, than with the prouder expectation of multiplying and varying the fources of inftruction, writes his

book

book after his own way; and takes his plates, perhaps, where he is directed by his bookfeller, or where he may moft fafely fteal; and often chufing them of a fafhion fifty years older than that book, into the gaps and interftices of which, they are to be nitched and ftuck up, wherever they will make the handfomeft figure, not where they will be of the moft ufe.

This ironical praife may be very fafely given to the older anatomifts for their love of original drawings, that having once fet their tafte to one certain fyftem of plates, they have been very conftant and true to their firft choice. It is thus that the plates of Vefalius, Fallopius, or Euftachius, have defcended, with fome diftortions and abridgements indeed, but ftill unpolluted with any ftain of originality, nor vitiated by any one improvement of reprefentation or of thought, through the books of Vidus Vidius, Pareus, Stephanus, Blanchardus, Veflingius, Riolanus, Verhein, Palfin, Dionis, and a thoufand others. Thus have the once beautiful plates of Vefalius, (mangled and deformed, cut down to fuit books of all fizes, twifted and accommodated to all fubjects and all forms of explanation,) defcended to us in fuch diftorted fhapes, that while we are looking over their books to fix upon them this indictment of plagiarifm, we can hardly recognife the original drawings fo fairly as to prove the deed.

Even

Even in the firft invention of our beft anatomical figures, we
fee a continual ftruggle between the anatomift and the painter;
one ftriving for elegance of form, the other infifting upon accuracy of reprefentation.   It was thus that the celebrated Ti-
tian confented to draw for Vefalius : Though it is but too plain
that there can be no truth in drawings, thus monftroufly
compounded betwixt the imagination of the painter, and the
fober remonftrances of the anatomift, ftriving for accurate anatomy, where the thing cannot be ; for thofe figures, which are
fuppofed to be drawn truly from the anatomical table, are
formed from the imagination of the painter merely ; fturdy
and active figures, with a ludicrous contraft of furious counte-
nances, and active limbs, combined with ragged mufcles, and
naked bones, and diffected bowels, which they are bufily employed in fupporting, forfooth, or even demonftrating with their
hands.   This vitious practice of drawing from imagination merely is well examplified in this, that anatomifts have, with one confent, agreed to borrow the celebrated Torfo for putting their
bowels into, to explain them there ; a practice which has defcended from the time of Vefalius down to Cheffelden, and from him
to the fyftems of the prefent day.

No painter in natural hiftory, in botany, in mechanics, nor in
any thing that relates to fcience, would dare to draw without

his

his subject immediately before him: but anatomists, who most of all need this clearness and truth, have been most of all arbitrary and loose in their methods; not representing what they saw, but what they themselves imagined, or what others chose to report to them:—hence the careless copying from book to book, the interpolations of anatomists, the interference of painters in a subject degrading to their higher art, the errors and mistakes of engravers, and the subjection of true anatomical drawing to the capricious interference of the artist, whose rule it has too often been to make all beautiful and smooth, leaving no harshness nor apparent blurr in all his work. Even the celebrated book of Albinus has been thus abused; and though he is sparing of cellular substance, and glands, and fat, and vessels; of all that gives a drawing its likeness to the human body; even the little that he had given, is now rounded down into the smoothness of ivory, as if a model had been made and drawn from. Albinus, (naturally sparing of ornament, and wanting in the natural character of parts) lived to see his drawings thus robbed of the little that they possessed of grace or nature; and then produced, as if in mere wantonness and sport, under the high title of ANATOMY of PAINTING; but by one, who seems too grave to have intended any stroke of irony, so refined as this.

A higher taste prevails in the present age; and the splendid and noble works of Morgagni, Haller, Bidloo, and Albinus, and

of

of Cheffelden, Hunter and Cowper, are drawn truly, and from
nature, and cannot be forgotten, while anatomy, and the arts de-
pending on it, continue to be efteemed.   Yet even, among thofe
great men, we have feen an idea gradually improving, till at laft
it was brought by Haller to the true point.   For Albinus's drawings are merely plans: Bidloo's tables are beautiful and mafterly;
but being wanting in regularity and order, they want altogether
the clearnefs of a plan; Haller's drawings are as fair as Bidloo's, as
regular as thofe of Albinus; and combine in one the truth and
fometimes the elegance of drawing, with the plainnefs and accuracy
of a mere plan.

If an anatomift fhall fet up a fkeleton, and draw it in poftures refembling thofe of life; if he fhall diffect the human body, ftudying and drawing it in parts; if he fhall continue drawing mufcle after mufcle, and one part after another, till he have
gone through the whole; if he fhall proceed then to take thefe drawings and notes of individual parts, and lay them over his firft
drawings of the bones; if he fhall try to match the parts belonging to fifty individual bodies of different fizes, of various forms,
dying, fome fuddenly, and others flowly, fome full and mufcular,
others emaciated and poor; what will the refult of all this be, but a
mere plan? It is a plan merely, through all the procefs, and in all
its parts; it cannot be other than a plan when the whole work is
                                                      accomplifhed

accomplished and set up. It was an unlucky theory of this
kind that carried the great ALBINUS, for fifteen years, through a
course of laborious diffections, painful and useless to himself;
but useful to all those who have to follow him: Still each
drawing of his is but a mere plan, resembling no individual
body, resembling in nothing the general drawing of the body; it is
such a view as never is to be seen in a diffection. It is not, like our
COUPER's nor like BIDLOO's, a true drawing of muscles dashed
with touches of glands, and fat, and cellular substance, which are
the natural diftinctions of parts; nor mixed with the branchings of
arteries or nerves, the chief objects for which we study the muscles;
but it is like a statue anatomised, where all the irregularities of substance, all the gradations of bones, ligaments, tendons, and flesh,
are rounded down with a studied smoothness; it is a figure which
the student can never compare with the body as it lies before him
for diffection; it is a figure suiting more the eye of the painter
than the eye of the anatomist; nor even pleasant to his eye, since
it stands in attitudes, which no swelling of particular muscles
seems to support.

In the other extreme is BIDLOO; for, in his plates, the master-
hand of the painter prevails almost alone; while whole sheets of
infinite labour serve only to explain the joinings of the clavicles, or
perhaps the form of one trifling muscle or gland. The formal fi-

b

gures of ALBINUS are more defireable than thefe. But, in either book,
we regret either extreme; in ALBINUS we think that we underftand every mufcle of the human body! but our knowledge hardly
bears the teft of diffection; the drawings and the fubject never can
be directly compared:—In BIDLOO, we have the very fubject before us! the tables, the knives, the apparatus, down even to the
flies that haunt the places of diffection, all are prefented with the
main object of the plate; and thus we have perfect confidence in
the drawing; in which alfo the parts are laid out in a bold and mafterly ftile, fo that the dead fubject and the engraving can well bear
to be compared. But in BIDLOO there is often no claffification nor
arrangement, no breadth of parts, by which we can underftand a
whole limb; a thigh is prefented with no one marked point; neither
the haunch nor the knee are feen: His plates are all elegance in refpect of drawing; in refpect of anatomy, they are all diforder and
confufion; and one muft be both anatomift and painter to guefs
what is meant, how the limb is laid, and what parts are feen.

It is to HALLER that we muft give the palm; who having to do
with parts chiefly, and not with a whole, has feldom offended by
drawing a diffected body, after a living form; nor by planning and
dividing a living form into the parts of a diffected body; but has
given his drawings truly from the anatomical table; and with the
trueft drawing, has given, very often, all the diftinctnefs of a
plan.

Now

Now we should always remember that anatomy is to be learnt only by diffection*; diffection is the firft and laft bufinefs of the ftudent; and when drawings are made for his ufe, the body fhould be laid out, as he is to order it in diffection; the belly fhould be difplayed, as he can difplay it in his fubject; an arm fhould be fo drawn, that, when he diffects the arm of the fubject, it may fall naturally upon the table, exactly as he finds it in his book; and ftill the pofture of arms, and legs, and heads, fhould be preferved diftinct and clear: enough of the general figure fhould be kept to explain the pofture of parts; there fhould be kept up a natural correfpondence among the feveral drawings; and while the true anatomical drawing is delivered upon one plate, a plan, if it be required, fhould be added upon the next.

b 2   I

* If anatomy is to be acquired in this way only, then muft we underftand by a fchool of anatomy a fchool of diffection: Yet thofe who have had the happinefs of profecuting their ftudies in foreign univerfities, or in the London fchools, will hardly believe it, that there is at leaft one place of education much celebrated, and worthy to be fo, where the ftudy of anatomy is denied or profcribed.—Where not only it is not praifeworthy, but even dangerous to propofe diffections; where the man who may be fo bold as to do his duty in that moft important ftudy, fhall be traduced in filthy pamphlets, thruft officioufly, and with intentions not of the pureft kind, into the hands of every young man who comes to fchool. If I have felt this, it has been ftill in filence; till I now fpeak of it, not formally, but by chance; not with the mean thought of prefenting myfelf as a perfecuted man, nor of indulging a refentment which were loft upon fuch people, or upon fuch an occafion; but to make my acknowlegements to one, whofe generous conduct is not unknown; who is truly interefted in the honour and reputation of that univerfity to which he belongs; who is at once an honour and defence to it; and whofe fingle praife, (may I be allowed to fay what touches myfelf fo nearly,) " fhall outweigh a whole theatre of " others."

I know but too well that few will submit to learn anatomy, as they should do, by the dry reading of anatomical descriptions, and the tedious comparing of these with the subject, or with their plates; and there are very few, who have learned this useful truth, that they are to become acquainted with parts only by being masters of the whole. One proposes to himself to learn the bones only; another designs to attend chiefly to the joints; a third will study the arteries only, " for the arteries are of chief use to the surgeon;" another delights in studying the viscera, and is sorely disappointed if he fail to understand the brain; while anatomy absolutely is not to be studied in parts, but is one fair and continued circle, where such is the correspondence, and mutual connection of all the parts, that he who would know the muscles, must first study the bones; and he who would learn the blood vessels, and nerves, (which are indeed the most important to the surgeon,) must know the muscles thoroughly. It is according to the muscles, that all the other parts are to be described; for when we trace the course of a blood vessel, it is by pursuing its intricate wanderings among the muscles: it gives its first branch to one muscle, its second branch to another; it forks into two, under the belly of a third; it goes through the substance of a fourth muscle, or accompanies its tendon, or runs along the edge of its fleshy belly: So that in describing a great vessel, we mark its exit from the trunk of the body, its entrance into the arm-pit or groin, its course down the arm or thigh; the dangers, the wounds, the operations of each great artery or nerve, are recorded according to the parts which

their

their feveral branches fupply. And befides thefe confiderations, which cannot but have their weight, we muft not forget, that the wounds of the mufcles, the fprains of tendons, the rupture of ligaments, the collections under the general fafciæ or broad tendons of the limbs, are of themfelves fufficient and direct motives; the only ones, indeed, that need be affigned for teaching the anatomy of the mufcles with particular care.

Yet, labour it as we will, how poorly ought we to think of our own diligence, when we find Statuaries or Painters ftudying the anatomy of the human body, with a perfeverance and fuccefs which may well put us to fhame! Painters merely, who having no object fo important, nor fo interefting, as the injuries and accidents of the body, defire nothing more than to underftand its external beauty and its form.

The Greeks lived in the moft delightful countries of the world; the moft beautiful people; fometimes happy, and always free. Among them the arts grew and flourifhed, and were to all ranks the chief bufinefs and pleafure of life:—for moderation and fimplicity was in their dwellings, while all their riches were referved for fhows and feftivals, for adorning their native city, for the public ufe. Their temples, and ftreets, and halls were filled with reprefentations of a beauty, which never exifted but among that happy people, or lives now only in their works, the admiration and reproach of our laggard times.—They faw, in their public games, the lovely forms of

their

their youth moving in dignity and grace: For there were feen in mixed affembly ;—in their women, the pureft models of female beauty ;—in their young men, the grandeft difplays of the manly form; moving and in action; infpired by every noble emulation, exulting in their ftrength; or advancing into the public view, only to fhow the beauties of their form.——Their artifts needed no helps of anatomy; but in thofe delightful fpectacles collected all the modes and forms of beauty, to combine them into one high ideal form. *

The moderns have come poorly after, in this great career; copy-ing coldly thofe half-animated forms, which are feen in our fchools of the arts fixed in laborious poftures, " felling their igno-" ble beauty for a price." Senfible of this great defect, our artifts have taken the help of anatomy to correct this tame unmeaning form; ftudying with a noble perfeverance, (but as their own critics acknowledge to us,) with but poor fuccefs. They ftudy each muf-cle; they note down its direction and ufe; they guefs at its office, and power in certain poftures of the body; and try to mark it in its juft place. The modern ftatuary, is like one wandering a-mong the ruins of fome noble city, who finding the remains of a temple, traces its lines among the ruins, and, upon this flender knowledge, tries to imagine and coldly reprefent to us its loft form and antient grandeur.

It

* " We are taught by philofophy, the natural pre-eminence and high rank of fpecific ideas " above individual forms."——HARRIS.

It was thus that Michael Angelo ſtudied our profeſſion : and ſtudied it ſo, that the leſſons of that great maſter are a reproach to thoſe who profeſs anatomical knowledge. His knowledge of anatomy gave to all his works a caſt " approaching more nearly to " the Etruſcan ſtyle, than to the purer taſte of the Greeks ;" marking them too harſhly with traits of learning. His violent diſtortions and ſudden ſhortenings of the limbs are leſs pleaſing to thoſe who delight in the delicate and higher beauty; fitting him leſs for repreſenting the female form, than for giving bold and terrible pictures of action and ſtrength. But ſtill he is correct and true in all that belongs to the anatomy of the human body ; and his ſtudies are a trial of the anatomiſt's ſkill;—for in looking upon one of theſe, we find that the knee, the ancle, the neck, the wriſt, each head and projecting point of bone, is truly marked; while the diſtortion of the figure, the violent action of the limbs, the ſhortenings and bending of the joints, and the intricacy of the whole poſture are difficult in the extreme; but ſtill each limb is true, and every individual muſcle ſwelling in its juſt degree, ſo as to preſerve correctly the proportions and balance of the whole. Should not we be aſhamed to compare our languid endeavours with the perfect knowledge of this great painter, the very notes of whoſe deeper ſtudies in anatomy we are unable to read ?

But in our profeſſion, though the very ſcience might almoſt be defined a knowledge of parts, induſtry and knowledge are but of low

2   repute,

repute, and the very name of diligence and mere labour, a term of
reproach; while genius is in truth nothing but a ftrong defire of
knowledge, and the fpirit of induftry its trueft mark. Let not
the ftudent of anatomy defpife labour, nor hope to acquire his
knowledge by other means. In juftice to his own genius, he
muft take all advantage of defcriptions, and drawings, and diffections, and plans; feeling, no doubt, in his firft difficulties the need
of every help, but ftriving to mount, by flow degrees, from fuch
elementary books, as that which I now prefent him with, to thofe
noble and fplendid works, which were the beginning of correct anatomy, and will not be forgotten, while that branch of knowledge is
refpected or known. And here may I not complain, that, in fche-
ming thefe plates, I am curbed and bound in by the oeconomy of my plan? If, indeed, by wifhing merely, the thing could be
accomplifhed, this word oeconomy fhould never more be heard of
in all that relates to fcience; but many are to ftudy our profeffion
who cannot command thofe noble works; and every young man
who is to ftudy an art in which the interefts of fociety are fo im-
mediate and fo ftrong, fhould have the means of inftruction put
within his reach. If there be any teacher, then, who being cir-
cumfcribed in point of time, would confent to offer his help and
inftructions in that form in which he could give them, regarding
more his duty than his good name, to him this motive fhall be my
apology; it fhall be my apology to all thofe who can feel with me
a fincere defire to do good and to be ufeful;—but not to all!—for
ftudents

students have been already warned, that they muft be jealous of thofe who pretend to give them plates; " that fome are capable of making plates for them, and fome are not ; that thofe who are beft able to give them plates, either will not undertake the labour, or cannot find time." And fo, the half only of this delicate argument was left unpronounced, which was already but too plain. Now, although fome unfortunate publifher of Anatomical Drawings was thus left impaled upon the horn of this broken dilemma, any implied reproach could not be aimed at me particularly, fince my book was not publifhed; it was only advertifed. This is perhaps a fort of caution, which it might in certain circumftances be very right, or very dutiful, or very convenient, perhaps, to give; as young men, no doubt, need fome careful perfon to inftruct and help their judgements, efpecially in fuch tender points as this is. But fhould it ever happen, that a man of high rank and character fhould be found, ftriving to hurt any poor endeavours of mine, I might feel that rifing within me, which it were almoft a meannefs to fupprefs *; and reply to him in the words of Lord Shaftfbury : " You, Sir, have a cha-" racter, which fets you above us far, and releafes you " from thofe decorums, and conftraining meafures of beha-

" viour

---

* Ille fapit, qui te fic utitur, omnia ferre

Si potes ac debes.   JUVENAL.

" viour, to which we of an inferior fort are bound; you may

" liberally deal out your compliments and falutations in what lan-

" guage you think fit; for I fhall but ftrive with myfelf to fup-

" prefs whatever vanity might naturally arife in me for fuch a fa-

" vour beftowed; for, whatever may in the bottom be intended by

" fuch treatment, it is impoffible for me to term it other than a fa-

" vour, fince there are certain enmities which it will ever be efteem-

" ed an honour to have deferved *."

· The author furely will not be accufed of fuch want of tafte, and relifh for elegant drawing or engraving, as to hold thefe plates out as excelling in what is beautiful; yet, may he not hope, that they are not wanting in what is ufeful? They want that fize which gives fplendor to a grander work, and of courfe that propor-tion, which gives the full idea of the human body; they want that elegant drawing, and careful engraving, which fhould do any idea juftice, which is fo neceffary in delivering the minuter parts with character and truth; all is wanting that belongs to the idea of a grander work; an idea, which the author could not but feel, yet durft not indulge. But ftill he hopes they may be found fimple, in-

telligible,

---

* Perhaps it was fome fuch critic as this that contrived that great anatomical drawing, which either I fhould not have mentioned at all, or fhould have given fome fhort account of.—Indeed it is not eafy to deliver a fair hiftory of even the moft trivial improvement, and very fel-dom are we able to difcover by what happy chance an idea firft fprang up in the mind of

its

teiligible, and plain ; having whatever belongs to a little fyftem of plates, intended merely to accompany a book of anatomy, and chiefly defigned for thofe who are entering on their ftudies, and but little advanced; and he trufts that he will be indulged, in trying fairly, whether by attending to the correfpondence of ideas and reprefentations, whether by ordering his drawings fo as to fuit his book, whether by a careful combination of defcriptions, drawings, and plans, he fhall not be able to deliver a fyftem of anatomy, intelligible, or perhaps eafy for his pupils; enabling them to enter the diffecting room with confidence, and to leave it, not without inftruction; and qualifying them alfo for underftanding thofe illuftrations, which he fhall continue to give, or the corrections and remarks of other teachers :—for that ftudent has but a mean idea of the value of his profeffion, who does not feek all means of inftruction ; and the teacher muft have a poor conceit of his prefent knowledge, who does not hope, by his own diligence, to correct himfelf; or to receive leffons from others, fometimes friendly, too often, in this world tinctured with its enmities and paffions ; fuch as are not pleafant in receiving, which ftill it is a duty to receive.

its author ; but perhaps the hiftory of this grand figure might go in the following terms. The ingenious Mr Cruikfhanks, with the defign of explaining all that he or Dr Hunter had injected, of the lymphatic fyftem, in one confiftent view, took a delicate and elegant drawing of the human body, and laid his lymphatics upon it, explaining at the fame time his intention, and making his apologies for this little plan ; but he could not forfee that the idea thus firft fuggef-

ted

WHILE I have ventured to fpeak fo fully concerning the general
defign of thefe plates, it is very natural for me to fay alfo a few
words concerning the mechanical labour.

I have drawn my plates with my own hand. I have engraved fome of
thefe plates, and etched almoft the whole of them: Which I mention only
to fhow, that they have their chance of being correct in the anatomy, and
that whatever, by my interference, they may have loft in elegance, they
have gained, I hope, in truth and accuracy.—And while I mention this, I
muft not be ungrateful to Mr Beugo, whofe fkill will, I hope, be fhown on
fome higher occafion, and whofe character muft not be hurt by any thing
that may be feen here ; for wherever in thefe plates all is fair and clean, it
is owing to his care ; and thofe blots of execution which are not fairly covered, have not come through his correcting hand.—Whatever he has done
alone has been hurried, allowing no time for artful or laborious engraving,
though ftill all that is here, I hope, is correct and true.

I

ted was to receive, in paffing through a greater mind, a grander form.—The expedient was tried
again, and the fecond anatomift refolving to outdo at one ftroke all his rivals, and knowing of no
furer way than this, had an engraving made of a moft gigantic fize ! An Afkapart ! A figure of full
fix feet in height ; which (bating the clumfinefs of conception) has turned out to be a drawing
of fuch fingular beauty, that it will not be rivalled; and as there can be no reprefentation of the
human body of more than 6 feet high, it pofitively cannot be excelled.—All thofe who underftand
the intention and effect of engraving, or who have any idea of the bold and free manner which
clafs drawings require, muft wonder even at the report of fuch a thing ; but not as our poet
Young wonders, " for wonder is involuntary praife ;" if the emotion be involuntary, it will moft
likely be of another kind.

I have endeavoured, alſo, to keep the explanation of theſe plates to the moſt ſimple and natural form; knowing, by long experience, that anato-mical deſcriptions are, even to the moſt earneſt and diligent ſtudent, very tedious and hard to be underſtood. The loading of ſuch a ſtudy as Anatomy with peculiar or affected language, and with needleſs terms of art, where too many are really needful, has a tawdry and vulgar appearance, of which we have much reaſon to be aſhamed; it is a barbarous jargon, to which our ear is ſubdued only by long and inveterate cuſtom: and our continual uſe of this traſhy language in ſchool books, preſents to the ſtu-dent the difficult and harraſſing taſk of learning at once a new ſcience and a ſtrange language.

Swift, who commends ſimplicity of language, and enforces his leſſon by the moſt beautiful examples, ſays, " When the water is clear you will " eaſily ſee to the bottom;" but anatomiſts have ſtirred up their techni-cal terms ſo thick, that the ſtudent has but a poor chance of ſeeing to the bottom, unleſs we ſhall agree in letting this ſediment quietly ſubſide a-gain.

The medical ſtudent is, indeed, ſo accuſtomed to hard words, that he can ſcarcely think any book accurate or complete that is without them; and however well he may underſtand its deſcriptions, cannot believe them true. He is not only accuſtomed to know the moſt difficult parts by the hardeſt names, but to have the detail given to him in ſuch expletives, as the Poſterior, Anterior, Superior, Inferior *; and often after all, this Superior Anterior portion

* Our ſcience in this country has got this vile farrago, of Anterior, Superior, &c. through bad tranſlations of Latin and French, where ſuch words as *Superieure* or *Superior* are in their place.

tion is but one extremity forfooth, or one portion of a part, which having other pofterior extremities, or anterior portions, has to pafs ftill through a long declenfion of thefe curious terms, which have not, like the terms in any other fcience, the property of conveying more regular and clear ideas, nor of faving fuperfluous words. They ftand in place of the fimple expreffion of upper or lower ends.—Now this clutter of hard names confounds the ear, as well as puzzles the judgement of the ftudent, and is truely a difgrace to the fcience ;—it looks as if we believed Anatomy to confift in ftrange terms, and that we could not write in true character of Anatomifts, but by departing as widely as poffible from the language of gentlemen. I have ventured, inftead of " fetting up this rank and file of tall opaque words " betwixt the reader's imagination, and my own conceptions," to make every defcription as fimple as may be,—ufing no hard words, but the pure names ; choofing rather that my book fhould be plainly underftood, than admired as a piece of unintelligible profound anatomy.

THE

FIRST BOOK

OF THE

BONES.

BOOK FIRST,

OF THE

BONES.

PLATE I.

This Plate explains the Text Book, from Page 35, to Page 52.

IN this Plate are reprefented the Adult and Fœtal Sculls, that they may be fairly compared with each other;——and there is explained here, not the minute anatomy of the individual parts, but the general view only, viz. the Bones of which the Cranium is compofed;——the Sutures by which the feveral bones are joined. And, in the Fœtal Scull, the form and procefs of Offification; and the interftices called Fontanelles, which are always left membraneous, during the flow offification of the child's head.

A   FIGURE I.

FIGURE I.

THE ADULT SCULL.

A   THE FRONTAL BONE, where (*a*) fhows the ferrated edge which forms the Coronal Suture; —— (*b*) the flatter part behind the Eye, which is plain and hollow for lodging the Temporal Mufcle; —— (*c*) is the acute angle of the bone, which is·called the External Angular Procefs, from its forming the outer angle or corner of the eye; ——and (*d*) is that prominence over the nofe, under which there is a fmall cavity within the bone, called the Frontal Sinus, which the furgeon avoids in performing the operation of trepan; though it is rather from the difficulty of perforating this part that he fhuns it, than from any danger in the perforation.

B   The PARIETAL BONE. The letter B points to that great line, which running according to the length of the bone, with a rainbow-like arch, divides the furface into two equal parts, of which the upper and fmooth-part (*e*) is covered with the thin expanded tendon of the OCCIPITO-FRONTALIS MUSCLE, while the lower part (*f*) has its furface radiated; and thefe radii are the impreffions of the particular bundles of which the Temporal Mufcle confifts; fo that " the white " femicircular line (B) reprefents the origin of the temporal mufcle; and the con- " verging lines on the furface (*f*) exprefs the manner, in which the fibres of " the mufcle are gathered into a fmaller compafs to pafs under the jugum." *Vid. P.* 61.—(*g*) points to a fmall hole in the back part of this bone, which is fometimes large, fometimes wanting; and which gives paffage to a fmall vein of the integuments, (going inwards to the longitudinal finus or great vein of the head) and alfo to a fmall artery, which accompanies the vein: (*h*) marks that corner which, running down fharper and longer into the temple, is often

     2   called

called the Spinous Procefs of the Parietal Bone; and this corner is the more to
be obferved, that it is under it that the great artery of the Dura Mater runs.

C   The OCCIPITAL BONE, of which but a very fmall part is feen in this direction.

D   Is the TEMPORAL BONE, feen full and direct from one fide; where (*i*) marks
that thin upper edge, which forms the fquamous future; (*k*) the deep and flat
part of the bone, on which the temporal mufcle lies; (*l*) the Maftoid or Mamillary Procefs, named from its refemblance to a nipple; (*m*) the Styloid Procefs,
which ftands out over the back part of the throat to give origin to feveral mufcles of the throat and tongue; (*n*) is the Zygomatic Procefs, which, joining
with a fimilar procefs of the cheek bone, forms the zygoma or arch; (*o*) marks
the Ring of the Meatus Auditorius Externus, or outward ring of the ear; and
(*p*) fhows a fmall hole, which, like that of the parietal bone, tranfmits a vein
paffing from without into the great finus or vein within the fcull, and which belongs fometimes to the temporal, fometimes to the occipital bone, or fometimes
is in the future betwixt them.

E   The OS MALAE, or bone of the cheek, which forms the lower and fore part
of the focket for the eye, and fupports the cheek; and by its prominence or
flatnefs gives the form of the face;——one procefs (*q*) is feen here going up
to meet the angular procefs of the frontal bone, and fo is named the Angular Procefs of the Cheek Bone; while (*r*) another procefs, called the Zygomatic Procefs
of the Cheek Bone, goes to meet the zygomatic procefs of the temporal bone,
forming the complete jugum, or yoke, under which the temporal mufcle paffes;
and from that prominent part of the cheek bone, which is marked (*s*), there go
two remarkable mufcles, one the Maffeter or Grinding Mufcle, which paffes from

this part of the cheek bone into the angle of the lower jaw to pull it upwards;
while another, a very slender and delicate muscle, goes from the same point
inwards towards the angle of the mouth, and is called Zygomaticus, or Distor-
tor Oris.

F   Points to the small bones of the Nose, named NASAL BONES; for there are
two of them forming the root of the nose, and the left one is seen here; the
small letter (t) points to what is called the Lateral Nasal Suture, which stretches *unites it*
to the upright process of the upper jaw bone.

G   Points to the UPPER JAW BONE, of which scarcely any thing is seen in this
view, except the circle called the Alveolar or Socket Process, in which the teeth
are set.

H   Marks the LOWER JAW BONE; and the letter is placed upon that point of the
Bone which is called the Angle, into which the Masseter Muscle is fixed;——
(u) marks that process of the jaw which is called Coronoid or Horn-like,
which goes up under the Zygoma to receive the great temporal muscle as it
passes under the arch;—— and (v) is the Condyloid Process, or that branch of the
lower jaw bone, which is crowned with the condyle or head, forming the joint or
hinge upon which the jaw moves; which head of the jaw bone is felt by putting
the finger before the flap of the ear.

THE SUTURES ARE,

1.   The CORONAL SUTURE, running across the head, joining the frontal to the parietal
bones, extending from ear to ear; and going down into the Temple, where it joins
the Squamous Suture, and, like it, is scaled, (i. e.) wants the indentations of a regular suture.

                                                    2. The

2. The LAMBDOIDAL SUTURE, joining the occipital to the parietal bones; ftriding over the occiput, refembling the Greek letter Δ.—But the refemblance is a little hurt by the accident of an Os Wormianum, or irregular bone, fuch as is found more frequently in this future than in any other; fometimes fingle, as in the fcull from which this was drawn; but fometimes in great numbers, and not unfrequently of the fize of a crown piece; thefe Offa Wormiana may difplace the Lambdoidal Suture fo, that being out of the ufual direction, it may be miftaken for a fracture.

3. The SAGITTAL SUTURE, joining the parietal bones to each other; extending from the Lambdoidal to the Coronal Suture, as an arrow lies betwixt the ftring and the bow.

4. The TEMPORAL or SQUAMOUS SUTURE, belonging chiefly to the temporal bone; and called fquamous or fcaled, becaufe the edges of the temporal and parietal bones are there extremely thin, and are laid over each other like the fcales of armour. One part marked (w) lying betwixt the occipital and parietal bones, is named the Additamentum Suturæ Squamofæ, or fupplement of the Squamous Suture.

5. Marks a part of the SPHÆNOIDAL SUTURE, joining the wing of the Sphænoid Bone, to the temporal, frontal, and parietal bones, for, in this hollow under the zygoma, all thefe bones meet by thin fcaled edges, and lap over each other; fo that all the futures in the Temple are fquamous.

6. The TRANSVERSE SUTURE, is one which runs acrofs the face, through the middle of the orbits, and over the root of the nofe, and the end of it appears here, joining the angular proceffes of the frontal bone, and of the cheek bone.

7. The ZYGOMATIC SUTURE.

FIGURE II.

FIGURE II.

THE FŒTAL SCULL.

EXPLAINS the FŒTAL SCULL;——where we find the holes, proceſſes, and other marks, very imperfect: Of courſe a ſhorter and more ſimple explanation will ſerve.

A Is The FRONTAL BONE; and the letter is ſo placed, as to mark the central point, where the oſſification begins; the oſſification being more perfect at this point, and going in a radiated form towards all the edges of the bone, leaves the oſſification very imperfect all round the edge of the bone; and at (*d*) there is a difference betwixt this and the Adult Scull, for here the cavity of the Frontal Sinus is not yet formed.

B The PARIETAL BONE; where alſo the letter marks the center of oſſification; the radii are very plain; and the edges are ſeen imperfect and membraneous, leaving all the ſutures imperfect. The ridge, which divides the bone, is not yet formed; for the Temporal Muſcle has not yet begun to mark the bone.

C The OCCIPITAL BONE; where the letter again in this bone, points to an oſſifying central point.

D The TEMPORAL BONE; where many parts, marked in the Adult Scull, as the Styloid and Maſtoid proceſſes,—the ſmall hole,—and the marks of the Temporal Muſcle, are all wanting. And the ring (*o*) of the Meatus Auditorius Externus,

is

is merely a ring; is fixed to the bone only, and not joined with it; and is here feen covered with the fmooth Membrane of the Tympanum, or Drum of the Ear.

E The CHEEK BONE; which, like all the other bones, is very round, and its edges blunt and ill defined.

F The SMALL BONES of the Nofe.

G The UPPER JAW BONE; where, fince the teeth are not yet come up, the Alveolar or Socket Procefs is not formed, nor even marked.

H The LOWER JAW BONE; where alfo the Alveolar Procefs is wanting, and where the branch of the jaw bone does not rife from the bafis, or lower line, with a bold and acute angle, but goes obliquely off, more horizontal, and more in the fame direction with the reft of the bone.

And laftly, the chief point to be obferved, in the fcull of a child, is the openings of the head; for the parietal bone is fo incomplete round all its edges, that it leaves all the futures imperfect and membraneous, and leaves fome openings particularly large. (*aaaa*) mark the four corners of the greater opening upon the top of the head; which, from the hypothefis of its ferving as a drain, is called the Fontanelle, or Fountain of Moifture. It has four angles, is formed by four croffing futures; the Sagittal Suture, defcending quite to the nofe. The Fontanelle is covered only with a thin and delicate membrane; it is named the Greater Anterior, or True Fontanelle, the opening of the head.

(*b*) Marks

(*b*) Marks a lesser opening, which is formed by the meeting of the Lambdoidal and Sagittal Sutures; but, as they do not crofs, there are here but 3 converging lines; three angles or points of bone; no perceptible opening, but the bones rather lapping over each other. It is over this point that the hair turns in a fort of vortex, if we may be allowed to explain it fo; and though the greater Fontanelle was thought to prefent in labour, this back Fontanelle is the true prefenting point.

(*c*) Marks a fmall Fontanelle, or membraneous interftice before the ear; and

(*d*) Marks another fmall Fontanelle behind the ear, in the place of the Additamentum Suturæ Squamofæ; and it is the more to be remarked, as it is through this little Fontanelle, that the accoucheur opens the head in the rare coincidence of preternatural pofture of the child, and deformed Pelvis; where after delivering the body, it is impoffible to get the head out: and he prefers this opening, and fhuns the back Fontanelle, left, in piercing there, he fhould cut the ligament of the neck, and fo lofe his hold of the head.

PLATE   II.

I

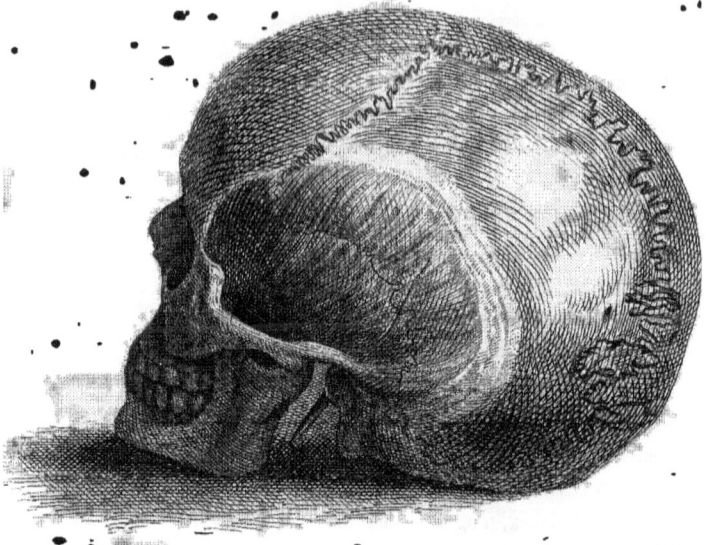

II

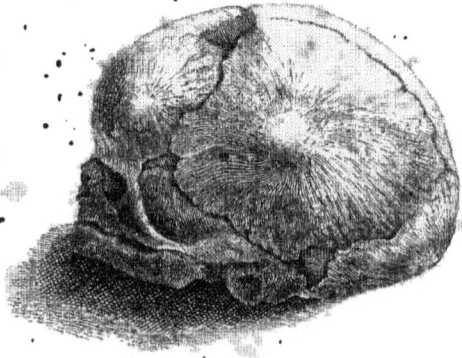

Published for the author Bell october 1794

I

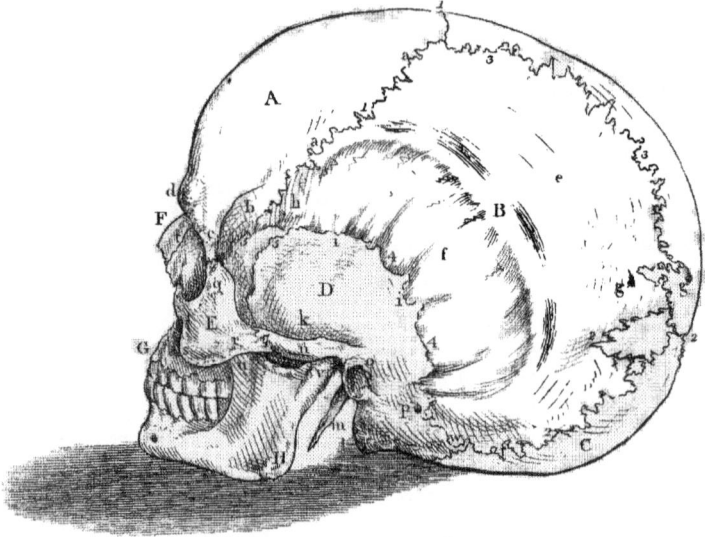

II

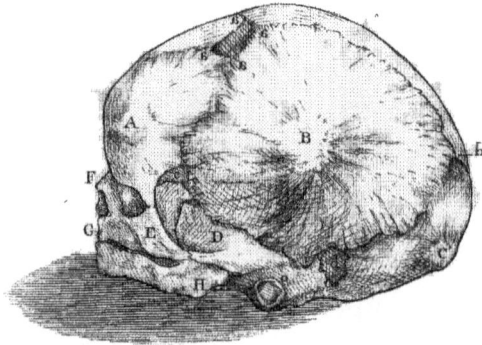

Engraved by Bell

P L A T E II.

This Plate explains the Text Book, from Page 52, to Page 65.

EXPLAINS the individual bones of the CRANIUM, the FRONTAL, PARI-ETAL, and OCCIPITAL BONES.

FIGURES I. AND II.

EXPLAIN the Os FRONTIS, or bone of the forehead. The numbers apply equally to either figure; and every number wanting in the firſt figure, muſt be ſought for in the ſecond.

1. The SUPERCILIARY RIDGES, on which the eye brows are placed, and which form the frontal ſinuſes. The ſkin is very firmly attached to the bone, all along this ridge; and the Frontal Muſcles ariſe here. The many ſmall dots, which are ſeen all along this ridge, are the marks of many little arteries, entering here to nouriſh the bone.

2. Points to that hole which is called the SUPERCILIARY HOLE, for it permits the ſmall Superciliary Artery and Nerve to come out from the ſocket of the eye to

B

tura

turn upwards upon the forehead, where they take the names of Frontal Artery and Nerve. On the one fide it is a fair round hole, on the other fide it is a notch only.

3. The two INTERNAL ANGULAR PROCESSES.

4. The two EXTERNAL ANGULAR PROCESSES.

5. The Hollow behind the External Angular Procefs, in which the Temporal Mufcle lies.

6. The NASAL PROCESS; ftanding up fharp and rough, betwixt the two internal angular proceffes.

7. The BUMP, at the inner end of the Superciliary Ridge, marking the place of the Frontal Sinus, and indicating alfo the fize of that cavity, by the degree of rifing.

8. The MOUTH of the FRONTAL SINUS; where it opens into the Nofe.

9. —is to be found on Figure II. only, and marks the SPINE, or Ridge to which the falx, or perpendicular partition of the Dura Mater is fixed; and (a) fhows the groove, in which the ridge very generally terminates.

10. The two ORBITARY PLATES; which are thofe two thin parts of the bone, which extend over the eye, fo as to form the roof for the eye, and the floor for the fore lobes of the brain; and it is by the continual preffure betwixt thefe two parts, that the Orbitary Proceffes become fo extremely thin, that they are quite tranfparent.

2   (b) Marks

(*b*) Marks the space or distance betwixt the two ORBITARY PROCESSES; which space is occupied by the Œthmoid Bone, which thus lies over the root of the Nose.

11. The mark of the Cartilaginous pully, through which the tendon of the Obliquus Oculi runs; and

12. Is the Superficial hollow for lodging the Lachrymal Gland in the upper part of the Orbit.

(*c*) Upon Figure II. shows the blind hole where the falx begins. This blind hole sometimes belongs to the Frontal Bone, sometimes to the Œthmoidal Bone, but lyes most commonly in the middle, betwixt the Œthmoid and Frontal Bones.

FIGURE III.

SHOWS the two OSSA PARIETALIA, or Parietal Bones, separated from the other bones of the Cranium, and also parted a little from each other, so as to show that serrated edge, which forms the Sagittal Suture.

1. Shows the serrated edges, forming the SAGITTAL SUTURE.

2. The edge of both bones, which, in a semicircular form, produce by their union with the Frontal Bone, the CORONAL SUTURE.

B 2

3. The

3. The thin femicircular edges, to which the Temporal bones are joined, forming the Temporal or SQUAMOUS SUTURE.

4. The SPINOUS PROCESS; or largeft and moft pointed corner of the Parietal Bone.

5. The RADIATED SURFACE, upon which the great Temporal Mufcle lies; (a) marking that ridge of the bone, which divides it into two parts, and beyond which the origin of the Temporal Mufcle does not extend.

6. The place where the Artery of the Dura Mater firft makes its impreffion, viz. at that fharp corner of the bone, which fhoots down into the temple.

N. B. The only hole, which belongs to the Parietal Bone, cannot be feen in this view, but is to be found in the firft plate.

—————

F I G U R E S IV. AND V.

EXPLAIN the Os OCCIPITIS. It is here fhown in two oppofite points of view, from within, and from without; the letters and figures apply to either figure; and the fourth figure naturally takes the lead, as the defcription of the Occipital Bone always begins with the external furface.

FIGURE IV. The outer furface.

1, The

1. The UPPER TRANSVERSE SPINE, formed for the implantation of the Trapezius and Complexus ; or produced, according to some, by the action of these great muscles.

2. The SMALLER and LOWER SPINE, formed by the Recti Muscles ; — small muscles which come up from the first Vertebra to lay hold on the Occiput.

3. The PERPENDICULAR SPINE, which divides the muscles of the opposite sides from each other ; and by this crossing, these two spines are named, in general terms, the Crucial Spines.

4. The Great TUBEROSITY, sometimes called the Spinous Process of the Occipital Bone. (a) The Cuneiform Process, which meets the Os Sphænoides. (b) The Condyle, or Joint Process, on which the head moves, at least in the nodding motion. (c) The Foramen Magnum, through which the spinal marrow passes out from the scull. (d) The Hole for the 9th, or Lingual, pair of Nerves. (e) The smaller Hole behind the Condyle, for the passage not of any nerve, but of a cervical vein going in towards the Great Lateral Sinus.

In FIGURE V. is explained the inner surface of the Occipital Bone ; and the figures are continued, that the description may go on still in the same order.

5. Is the ridge to which the Tentorium, or membrane which supports the brain, and defends the Cerebellum, is fixed.

6. The two furrows, in which lie the Right and Left Lateral Sinuses, making this broad groove.

7. The two hollows for lodging the backmost lobes of the brain, above the place of the Tentorium or supporting membrane.

2

8. Two

8. Two fimilar hollows, for lodging the two lobes of the Cerebellum, below the place of the Tentorium or crofs membrane.

9. The mark of a fmall falx or procefs of the Dura Mater ; which is like the great one, and like it contains a fmall finus or vein in it, the groove of which fmall finus is eafily feen here.

(*a*) The Cuneiform Procefs. (*c*) The Foramen Magnum. (*d*) The hole for the ninth pair of Nerves. (*f*) The hollow or thimble-like cavity, in which the end of the Lateral Sinus lies; for at this point the finus turns fuddenly round, efcapes from the fcull, and getting down into the neck, lofes the name of Sinus, and takes that of Internal Jugular Vein.

(*g*) There was left fticking to the end of this bone a fragment of the Sphœnoid bone, fo that at this point the Cuneiform proceffes of the Occipital and Sphœnoid bones are fo united, that to feparate them (in the adult at leaft), we muft break them ; and in breaking thefe bones, the great cell of the Spœnoid bone, or part of it, ftuck to the Cuneiform procefs of the Occipital bone ; and this cell is marked (*g*).

PLATE

I

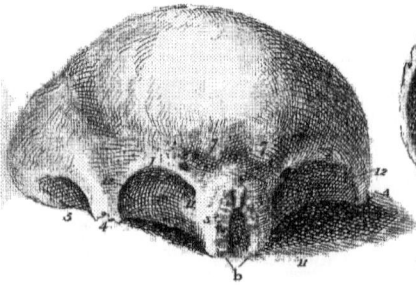

II

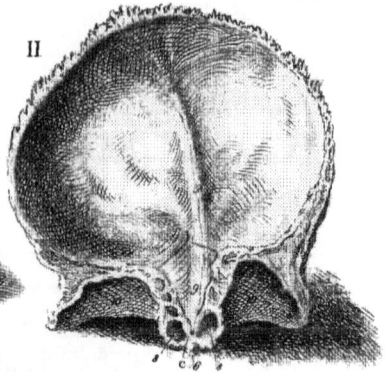

III

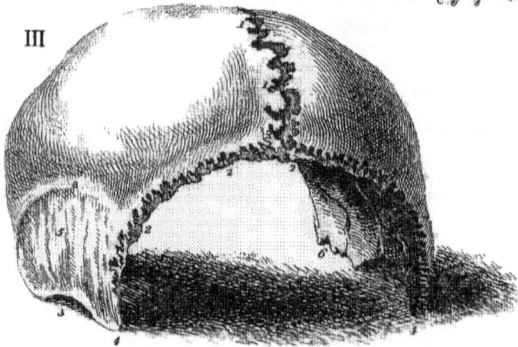

IV

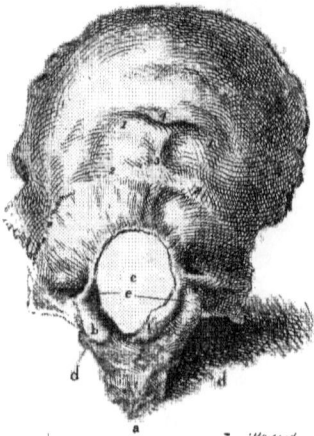

V

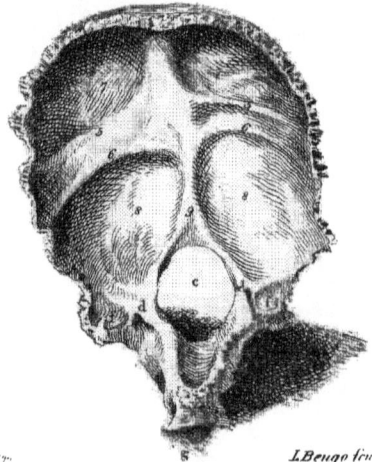

L.Bengo Sculp.

P L A T E   III.

This Plate explains the Text Book, from Page 65, to Page 94.

Explains much of the difficult Anatomy of the Scull; for thefe bones, the Temporal, Œthmoid, Sphoenoid, and Upper Jaw Bones, have many curious and intricate parts.

———

F I G U R E S   I.   and   II.

Explain the Temporal Bone; and now again the letters and numbers belong in common to both figures; to Figure I. which explains all the parts that are upon the outfide of the Temporal Bone, and alfo to Figure II. which explains all that fide of the Temporal Bone which is towards the brain.

The Great Divisions of the Temporal Bone, are; (a) The fquamous, or thinner part, forming the Squamous or Scaley Suture. (b) The Pars Petrofa, or Rocky Part, which is, indeed, in the child, a diftinct bone. (c) The Occipital Angle, or that corner of the bone, which is joined to the Os Occipitis, by the Additamentum Suturæ Squamofæ.

THE

THE PROCESSES F THE TEMPORAL BONE ARE,

1. The ZYGOMATIC PROCESS, ftretching forwards to meet that of the cheek bone.

2. The STYLOID PROCESS, ftanding downwards over the throat, to give origin to many of the mufcles of the throat.

3. The VAGINAL PROCESS, which is a kind of rough rifing at the root of the Styloid Procefs.

4. The MASTOID or MAMILLARY PROCESS, which is not formed in the child; which confifts of cells; it is felt immediately behind the ear, belongs to that organ, and is perforated (fo it is propofed at leaft) in certain kinds of deafnefs.

5. The AUDITORY PROCESS, which is named a procefs, becaufe it is in the child a diftinct part, and ftill is in the adult (as reprefented here) a prominent ring.

The HOLES of the TEMPORAL BONE relate chiefly to the EAR.

1. (d) Marks the MEATUS AUDITORIUS EXTERNUS, the outer Auditory hole, upon which the drum of the ear is braced down.

2. (e) The Internal Auditory Hole, or MEATUS AUDITORIUS INTERNUS, by which the Auditory Nerve has accefs to the Ear.

3. (f) A fmall hole for admitting a delicate thread-like nerve, which returns from
                                                                without

without into the Cranium again, and joins the Portio Dura, or hard part of the Auditory Nerve while it is going along the paffages within the Ear.

4. (g) The STYLO-MASTOID HOLE; which has its name, from its being at the root of the Styloid and Maftoid proceffes; it gives paffage to the Portio Dura, or that fmall hard Nerve, which accompanying the Auditory Nerve, goes along with it into the paffage of the Ear; but, while the Portio Mollis, or proper Auditory Nerve remains within the Ear, this Portio Dura, a diftinct Nerve, and deftined for the face, comes out by the STYLO-MASTOID HOLE, under the ear, and fpreads upon the cheek.

5. (h) Marks the ragged end of the Petrous Portion. The bony part of that canal, named the EUSTACHIAN TUBE ends here; but the Tube is chiefly Cartilaginous, and therefore in this the dried bone, its openings appear quite irregular and rough; and when the ftudent looks for the Euftachian Tube, he finds nothing but confufed and ragged openings. The mouth of the Euftachian Tube, as it appears when dried, is feen in its right place, *Vid. Pl.* VI.

6. (i) The hole for the CAROTID ARTERY is alfo to be looked for at this point, though it cannot be feen in this particular view, unlefs the end of the Petrous Portion were turned more directly towards the eye.

(k) Is the Great FURROW, which the Lateral Sinus, or great internal vein makes, forming a thimble-like cavity at (l), by the laft fudden turn which it makes before leaving the fcull.

(m) Is a very fmall FURROW, formed by a fmall Sinus, or vein, which goes along the ridge of the Petrous Portion.

C

7. (n) Is

7. (*n*) Is the laſt or 7th hole of the Temporal Bone. This is the ſmall hole, formerly mentioned for the paſſage of a trifling vein from without into the Lateral Sinus.

N. B. The joint or Condyle of the lower jaw is ſet in the hollow (*o*) juſt under the root of the Zygomatic Proceſs.

———

F I G U R E S III. AND IV.

EXPLAIN the ŒTHMOID BONE; FIGURE III. ſhowing chiefly the upper ſurface of the bone, which ſupports the fore part of the brain, and which is marked by the Criſta Galli (*b*); and FIGURE IV. ſhows that confuſed ſurface, which hangs over the root or upper part of the Noſe, and whoſe ſpongy bones, (*dd*) form a part of the Organ of Smell.

(*a*) The CRIBRIFORM PLATE is the center, as it were, of this bone, to which all the other parts are referred; this plate is perforated by the Olfactory Nerves, and it is from this horizontal and perforated plate, that the whole bone has its name.

The parts belonging to the Œthmoid Bone are,

1. (*b*) Is the Perpendicular Proceſs, which ſtands up from the Cribriform Plate, towards the brain; and is named CRISTA GALLI.

2. (*c*) Is the NASAL PLATE; which forms the Septum or partition of the Noſe, ſtanding perpendicularly downwards and forwards, as the Criſta Galli ſtands upwards: the Criſta Galli and the Naſal Plate, are exactly oppoſite to each other.

3. (*dd*) The

3. (*dd*) The two upper Spongy Bones; they are named spongy, from their constitution, for they consist of cells; they are called Ossa Spongiosa Superiora, to distinguish them from two similar bones, which hang in the lower part of the Nose. They are spoken of as distinct bones, while they are but parts of the Œthmoid Bone.

4. (*e*) The ORBITARY PLATE of the Œthmoid Bone; which, as it is inclosed among the other bones of the Orbit, seems to be a distinct bone surrounded by a peculiar future, and so is named the Os Planum; though it is merely the flat side of the Œthmoid Bone.

5. (*f*) Marks the place where the Os UNGUIS should be seen; but it is pulled away to show the numerous cells of the Œthmoid Bone. These cells are divided into two sets, one set attached to the Orbitary Plate, or flat square side of the Œth-moid Bone, the other set to the Spongy Bone.

6. (*g*) FIGURE IV. shows that set of the cells, which more particularly belongs to the Spongy Bone, and (*h*) FIGURE III. shows the cells opened from above, to give a view of those, which more particularly belong to the Orbitary Plate.

Whatever farther is necessary to the demonstration of the Œthmoid Bone, is to be found in Plates V. and VI. where the cells are particularly well explained.

———

FIGURE V. AND VI.

EXPLAIN the SPHOENOID, PTEREGOID, or WEDGE-LIKE BONE; it is named Pteregoid from its resemblance to a bat, and is so presented here, as to suggest the likeness.

Figure V. shows the back view of the bone, *viz.* that which is turned towards the skull;—Figure VI. shows the front view, *viz.* that which is connected with the bones of the face.

Its Processes are,

1. The ALAE, or wings, commonly named the Temporal Proceffes, for they lie in the Temples; the Temporal Mufcles lie upon them, and their upper edge is fquamous like the edge of the Temporal bone, and forms part of the Squamous Suture.

2. Marks that fmooth furface of this TEMPORAL PROCESS, which, being turned towards the eye, enters into the Orbit, and fo is named the ORBITARY Procefs of the Sphœnoid Bone.

3. The fmall and fharp SPINOUS PROCESS.

4. The hook-like point of the Spinous Procefs, which is often named the Styloid Procefs.

5. The External PTEREGOID PROCESSES; which are two flat and broad plates.

6. The two internal PTEREGOID PROCESSES; which ftand off a little higher, and more direct from the body of the bone; they are fmaller; and terminate in a little hook. The Pteregoid Mufcles, which go to the lower jaw, arife from the proceffes themfelves; and the TENSOR PALATI MUSCLE turns round this little hook.

7. The AZYGOUS, or fingle Procefs; which is fingle, becaufe it ftands out from the middle of the bone. It forms part of the partition for the Nofe, and is thence named NASAL PROCESS.

8. The

8. The two ANTERIOR CLYNOID PROCESSES.

9. The two POSTERIOR CLYNOID PROCESSES.

10. The fpace bounded by thefe four CLYNOID PROCESSES; which, from refembling a Turkifh faddle, is named, SELLA TURCICA.

11. The two little wings of Ingrafias, called the TRANSVERSE SPINOUS PROCESSES.

The cells, which occupy the body of this bone, lying under the SELLA TURCICA, are to be feen at (g) Figure VI. and again in Plate VI.

———

The HOLES proceed next in order, and are marked alfo with a fuit of numbers, that the demonftration may be continued and entire.

1. (a) The two OPTIC HOLES, tranfmitting the Optic Nerves; which are the fecond pair of the fcull; for the firft pair, viz. the Olfactory Nerves pafs through the Œthmoid Bone.

2. (b) The FORAMEN LACERUM; or wide hole, which permits the third, the fourth, the firft branch of the fifth, and the fixth pairs of Nerves to pafs; for all thefe are fmaller nerves, deftined for the Mufcles of the Eye, and enter thus at the bottom of the focket, while the fecond pair is the proper Optic Nerve.

3. (c) The FORAMEN ROTUNDUM; it tranfmits the fecond branch of the fifth pair which goes to the upper Jaw.

4. (d) Is

4. (*d*) Is the FORAMEN OVALE, (larger than the Foramen Rotundum) which tranfmits the third branch of the fifth pair, going to the lower jaw.

5. (*e*) The SPINOUS HOLE, the Foramen Spinale, which is a fmall hole in the very point or tip of the Spinous Procefs. It is not for the transmiffion of a nerve; but for the entrance of that fmall artery which belongs to the Dura Mater, and which goes along the inner furface of the Parietal Bone, marking it with its furrow. A briftle is paffed through this hole in one fide, to fhow the courfe of the artery.

6. The fixth Hole. The PTEREGOIDEAN, or VIDIAN HOLE, is not to be feen in this view; but is to be feen in the next Plate, IV. where it is marked with its proper number, 6.

(*f*) Reprefents the rough furface where the cuneiform or wedge-like part of this Sphœnoid Bone has been broken off from the wedge-like procefs of the Occipital Bone.

(*g*) Marks the Cells of the Sphœnoid Bone, which are occafionally very large, as in this Bone; and which make all the bone hollow under the Cella Turcica.

(*h*) Shows where the Palate Bone had adhered to the Sphœnoid;—and the Palate Bone, being torn away, has broken, and left fome of its fmall cells fticking here to the Sphœnoid Bone.

N. B. The Cells of the Palate Bone are explained in the next plate.

This Bone is connected;——at (*i*) Figure VI. with the Œthmoid Bone before;—at (*f*) Figure V. with the Os Occipitis behind;—at (1.) with the Temporal Bones in the Temples. The Spinous Procefs (3.) is locked in betwixt the Temporal and Occipital Bones;——

Bones ;—and the Pteregoid Proceſſes (5.) are joined to the Palate Bone, and form the back of the Noſtrils. *Vide* next plate, where the Pteregoid Proceſſes are ſeen in their place.

———— ———— ————

FIGURE VII. AND VIII.

THE VII. and VIII. figures of this plate explain the UPPER JAW BONE ; Figure VIII. ſhowing its Internal Surface, viz. that next to the noſe, with the wide opening of the Antrum, or Great Cavity of the Jaw. Figure VII. ſhowing the outſide of the Bone, explaining the outſide walls of the Antrum, or Great Cavity : ſo that, by comparing the two ſides of the bone, one can eaſily underſtand the great extent of the Antrum, or Cavity ; and how pulling a tooth will open the way for matter flowing out from it.

1. The NASAL PROCESS which riſes up on each ſide to form the ſides of the noſe. The Arch forms the ſides of the noſe ; and the rough pointed ending of this Naſal Proceſs is connected with the Os Frontis.

2. Is the ORBITARY PLATE, or that plate which forms the floor of the eye, and the roof of the Antrum, or Cavity.

3. The MALAR PROCESS, or that broad rough ſurface upon which the Cheek Bone reſts.

4. The

4. The ALVEOLAR PROCESS, or that projecting femicircle, which holds the teeth ; thence named Alveolar, or Socket Procefs.

5. The PALATE PLATE, or Procefs ; of which we fee the rough edge only, viz. that edge by which the Middle Palate Suture, the future in the roof of the mouth, is formed.

N. B. The Palate Plate is feen full in Plates IV. V. and VI.

6. The ANTRUM MAXILLARE, or HIGMORIANUM. This great cavity appears with a very wide opening here in the naked bone ; but this opening is covered in the entire fcull, both by the lower fpongy bone, and by the nafal plate of the palate bone. This nafal plate of the palate bone is left in this drawing covering a part of the Antrum ; the reft of this opening is naturally covered by a membrane, which leaves but one fmall hole..

The Nafal Plate of the Palate Bone which is left fticking upon the Antrum is marked (*a*).

(*b*) Marks the only Hole of the Upper Jaw Bone. It is named the Infra-Orbitary Hole. A chief nerve of the face comes out here, named (with its hole) the Infra-Orbitary Nerve.

The proper Infra-Orbitary Hole is marked (*b*) ; and the Canal by which the nerve comes down is marked (*c*) : at this place the nerve lies under the eye, upon the floor of the orbit,—making a very large groove and hole upon this Orbitary Plate of the Upper Jaw Bone ; for arteries running along bones do not make deeper grooves than the nerves do.

N. B.

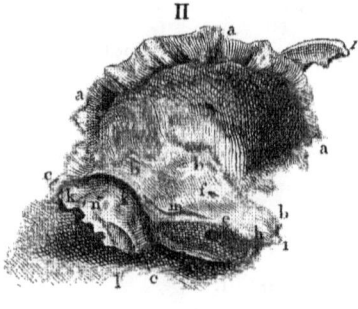

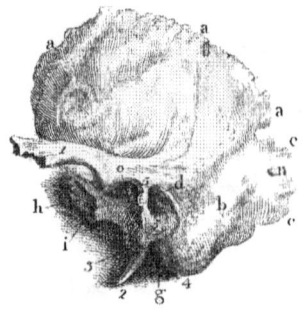

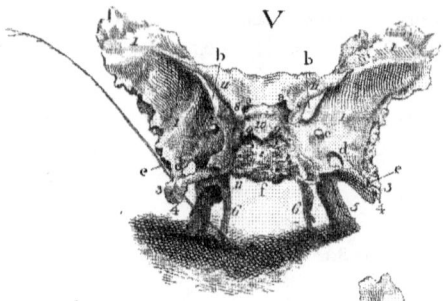

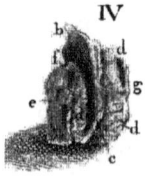

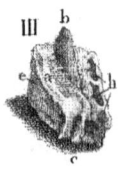

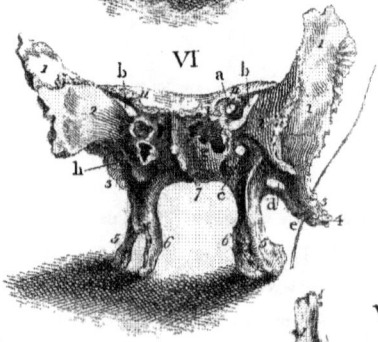

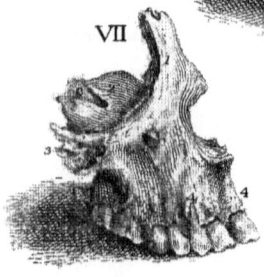

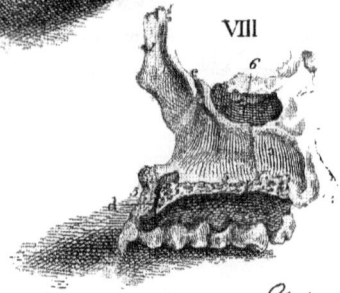

II

V

IV

III

VI

VII

VIII

Etched by J. Bell.

N. B. This Infra-Orbitary Nerve is a chief branch of the Superior Maxillary Nerve.

(*d*) Marks the Foramen Incisivum; fo named from its being juft above the Incifores or cutting teeth. It is alfo named Anterior Palatine Hole; it is complete only when the two jaw bones are joined, as in Plate IV. Fig. III. at (*l*) which marks this anterior Palatine hole.

(*e*) Marks the courfe of the Lachrymal Duct, or tube which conveys the tears, which, after having paffed through the Os Unguis, makes this groove in the Nafal Procefs of the upper jaw bone, and ends or opens into the Nofe juft where this duct ends.

D   PLATE

P L A T E   IV.

This Plate explains the Text Book, from Page 85, to Page 104.

EXPLAINS the BONES of the FACE, and the LOWER JAW BONE.

F I G U R E I.

REPRESENTS the two NASAL BONES, laid to each other in their natural direction; by which is explained,

1. The NASAL SUTURE; joining thefe two Nafal Bones to each other.

2. The SERRATED SURFACE, by which they are joined with the Os Frontis, at the roughnefs round the root of the Nafal Procefs; which union forms part of the Tranf-verfe Suture.

3. The ROUGH SURFACE, by which they are joined to the two cartilages that form the Alæ Nafi, or Wings of the Nofe.

4. The ROUGH SURFACE, by which they are fixed to the Nafal Proceffes of the upper jaw bone.

F I G U R E II.

EXPLAINS the Os UNGUIS, where both the drawings fhow that furface which appears in the orbit; and in both of them is feen,

1. The

1. The plain furface upon which the eye rolls; and

2. The Groove which holds the Nafal Duct.

FIGURE III.

EXPLAINS, by a ufeful drawing, many very important parts on the bafis of the
fcull. (*a*) the Foramen Magnum: (*b*) the Condyle: (*c*) the two Pteregoid Proceffes; (*d*) the Hook of the Inner Pteregoid Procefs, fhowing how the Tendon
of the Circumflex Mufcle may twift round it: (*e*) the Styloid Procefs: (*f*) the
Mamillary Procefs: (*g*) that part of the Palate, or roof of the mouth, which is
formed by the upper jaw bones: (*h*) the fmaller part of the Palate, formed by the
proper palate bones; (*i*) the Middle Palate Suture: (*k*) the Tranfverfe Palate Suture:
(*l*) the Anterior Palatine Hole, or Foramen Incifivum: (*m*) the two Pofterior Palatine
Holes, tranfmitting the nerves for the palate: (*n*) the Vomer, or bone forming the
feptum or partition which divides the two noftrils: (*o*) the two Upper Spongy Bones,
viz. thofe belonging to the Œthmoid Bone, hanging in their places high in the noftrils: (*p*) the two Lower Spongy Bones, which are independent bones hung by a
hook upon the fide of the Antrum Highmorianum, and confequently hanging very
low in the noftril.

FIGURES IV. V. AND VI.

EXPLAIN the PALATE BONES; where Figures IV. and V. fhow the two Palate
Bones feparated from each other, and from the other bones. Figure VI. fhows the
two Palate Bones joined. On thefe drawings, the fame figures ftill mark the fame
points,—the numbers marking Proceffes, and the letters running under them marking as ufual the leffer parts.

1. Shows

1. Shows the PALATE PLATE, or Procefs of the Palate Bones; and in FIGURE VI. the
palate plates are joined, fo as to form the back part of the middle palate future:
(q) is the broad rough furface by which the two palate bones are oppofed to each
other, and which forms the Middle Palate Suture: (r) is the middle point, from which
the Uvula, Pap, or Gurgulion hangs down.

2. Is the PTEREGOID PROCESS of the palate bones, having a little hollow into which the
Pteregoid Proceffes of the Sphœnoid Bone are received.

3. Is the NASAL PLATES, which lie within the noftrils; and which, by lying flat upon
the fides of the Antrum Highmorianum, clofe it in part.

4. Is the ORBITARY PROCESSES; for the Nafal Procefs lies up along all the fide of the
noftril, and ends in a broader knob, which enters into the focket of the eye at its
deepeft part, and is there named Orbitary Procefs.

5. Marks the Cell or Cells of the Palate Bone, which are in its Orbitary Procefs, and
which are joined to thofe of the Sphœnoid bone.

FIGURES VII. AND VIII.

T HE two SPONGY BONES.

FIGURE VII. Explains the rolled and fpongy appearance of the fpongy bone. It reprefents that furface which is turned outwards, i. e. towards the feptum of the nofe.

FIGURE VIII. fhows that flatter fide which is turned towards the Antrum Highmorianum, and clofes it; and the letter (s) marks the fmall point, or hook-like procefs, by which this lower fpongy bone is hung upon the edge of the opening into
the Antrum Highmorianum. (t) is the fore end of the fpongy bone, which is turned forwards in the nofe, covering the lower end of the nafal duct; fo that in
feeking to clear the duct with a probe, we muft pafs it under this point. (u) is
the other end of the fpongy bone, which is turned backwards in the noftrils.]

The

The pofition of the fpongy bone in the noftrils is well explained in Figure III. and the fore part of the fame fpongy bone is feen in Plate VI. Figure II.

FIGURE   IX.

REPRESENTS the VOMER.

1. The GROOVE, in its upper part, by which it fits aftride upon the Azygous Proceffes of the Œthmoid and Sphœnoid Bones.

2. Its Lower Groove by which it fits down upon the rifing point of the Maxillary and palate bones: and (r) Figure VI. fhows how it ftands upon the palate bones. The letter (v) Figure VI. fhows the Great Groove turned upwards to be fixed to the Azygous Proceffes of the Œthmoid and Sphœnoid bones, and the letter (n) Figure III. fhows the Vomer in its right place in the nofe, dividing the noftrils.

3. The Ragged Grooved Surface, which looks forwards and receives the plate of cartilage, which completes the partition betwixt the noftrils.

FIGURE   X.

REPRESENTS the CHEEK BONE.

1. Shows the Upper Orbitary Procefs.

2. Marks the Inferior or Lower Orbitary Procefs.

3. The Maxillary Procefs.

4. The Zygomatic Procefs; and

5. Marks the plate which forms the lower and fore part of the focket for the eye, and fo is named the Internal Orbitary Procefs.

2

FIGURES XI. AND XII.

Explain the lower jaw bone, in two views ; but every Figure applies to each bone, and the Figures proceed in the order of the Text Book.

1. The Chin ; the lines comprehend the Chin in their course, and they terminate so as to mark the small Mental Holes on both sides of the Chin, where the nerves, after having furnished the teeth, come out upon the face.

2. Marks the line of the Base of the Jaw, extending from the Chin to the Angle.

3. Marks the Angle of the Jaw, which is irregular and knotty, by the insertion of the great Masseter Muscle.

4. The Coronoid Processes of the jaw.

5. The Condoloid or Articulating Processes ; (*y*) the great hole which receives the lower Maxillary Nerve. We see here likewise the deep and wide groove that leads to the nerve ; and another deep, but smaller groove, which shows where the nerve which belongs to the tongue, departs from the great nerve, and runs along the inner side of the jaw bone betwixt it and the tongue.

6. Is the Alveolar or Socket Process, with the teeth in it.

PLATE

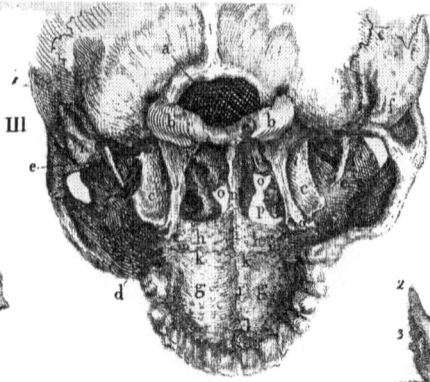

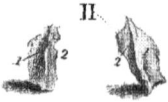

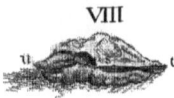

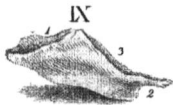

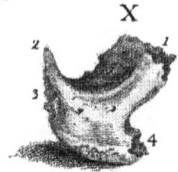

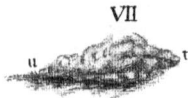

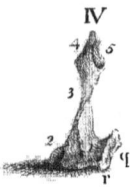

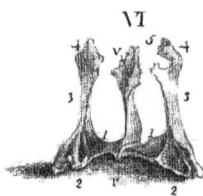

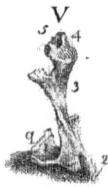

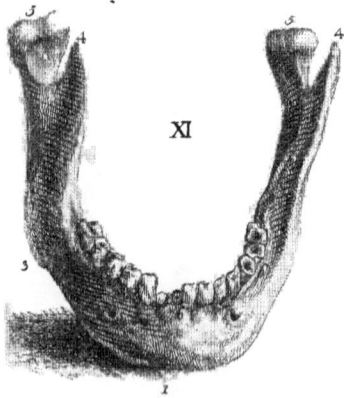

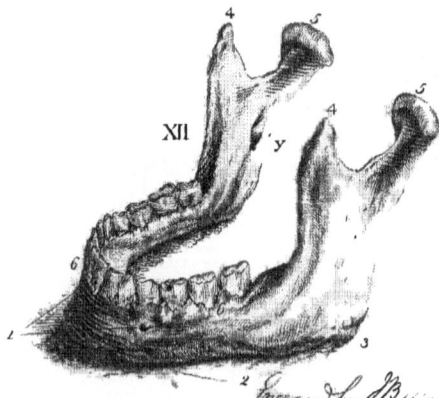

Published for the author J. Bell october 1794.

Engraved by J.B.

P L A T E   V.

This Plate explains the Text Book, in all the Chapters upon the Scull.

IS a general view of the CRANIUM,——explaining and connecting the demonſtrations of the individual parts.

F Í G U R E   I.

IN this view, where the Cranium or Scull Cap is cut off, and the baſis ſeen from within, the thing that firſt ſtrikes the eye is,—the formal and regular diviſion of the Cranium into three hollows (1. 2. 3.); and each of theſe is like a ſtage or deck, the one lower than the other.

(1.) Is the fore part of the baſis of the Scull, the ſhalloweſt and moſt ſuperficial hollow. It is formed chiefly by the Frontal, Œthmoidal and Sphœnoidal Bones. It is marked with undulating lines, correſponding with the inteſtine-like convolutions of the brain. ——This diviſion ſupports the Fore Lobes of the brain, and gives paſſage to the Olfactory and Optic Nerves.

(2.) Is a large hollow, cup-like, deeper than the firſt;——lying under the temple;—— formed chiefly by the wings of the Temporal and Sphœnoidal, and by the corners of the Frontal and Parietal Bones. This holds the Middle Lobes of the brain, contains the Petrous part of the Temporal Bone;—gives out all the ſmaller Nerves be-

E.   longing

longing to the Eye, and all the great nerves belonging to the Upper and Lower Jaws ; it gives alfo the Auditory Nerves, which enter here into the Petrous Portion of the Temporal Bone.

(3). Is a ftage lower ftill, being the deepeft hollow of the three ; is formed chiefly by the cup of the Occipital Bone, and by a fmall part of the Temporal Bones ;—and as the Cerebellum fupports the back lobes of the brain, this hollow may reprefent the back lobes, or the third divifion of the brain ;—fo this laft hollow con- tains the Cerebellum ; gives out the Lingual Nerves, which pafs through a hole of the Os Occipitis ; and fends out the Spinal Marrow through the Fora- men Magnum, or Great Hole.

FIRST DIVISION.

In the firft divifion are feen the parts and holes of the FRONTAL, ŒTHMOIDAL, and SPHOENOIDAL BONES.

FRONTAL BONE.

(a) Marks the Cancelli, or Diploe of the Frontal Bone fo cut as to make the Cancelli appear very wide ; but that proceeds from having cut the fcull very low, which has taken off the outer layer of the Orbitary Procefs. (b) Marks the regular or proper Frontal Sinufes, which are thus underftood to be like enlarged cells of the Diploe ; while (c) fhows a part of the cells going down into the Orbitary Plates : for the finufes fometimes extend thus all over the eye, as in this fcull ; and the letter (c), while it points to this extenfion of the Frontal Sinus, is fo placed as to mark the undulating forms, which the lobes of the brain give to this thin Orbitary plate of the Frontal Bone.

ŒTHMOIDAL

ŒTHMOIDAL BONE.

There is incafed betwixt (*c c*) the Orbitary Plates of the Frontal Bone, the Cribriform plate of the Œthmoidal Bone;—where (*d*) marks the Cribiform Plate with its numerous fmall holes for tranfmitting the Olfactory Nerves. (*e*) Marks the Crifta Galli, whence the Falx begins. (*f*) Points to that hole which is called the Blind Hole, which is as fmall as a pin's point, and which belongs in common to the Œthmoidal and Frontal Bones.

N. B. The fmall crack, to which the lines running downwards from (*d*) point, and which indicates the Suture furrounding the Œthmoidal Bone and named Œthmoidal Suture, can hardly be miftaken.

SPHOENOIDAL BONE.

The Sphenoid Bone is known here by its two procefles named TRANSVERSE SPINOUS, or LITTLE WINGS of INGRASIAS marked (*g*); the lines from the letter (*g*) point to the Sphœnoidal Suture, which feparates this Bone from the Frontal and Œthmoid Bones. (*h h*) Mark the two Anterior *Clinoid* Procefles. (*i*) Marks the Pofterior Clinoid Procefs; for it is rather one Procefs terminating in two little horns or knobs. (*k*) Is fet down in the Sella Turcica in the very centre of the Clinoid Procefles where the Pituitary Gland is lodged. (*l l*) Mark the two Optic Holes, which are fcarcely feen, for they lie under the two Anterior Clinoid procefles, fo as to be almoft hidden by them : —— The two lines going from the letter, (*m*) mark the two wide grooves, which are formed by the Carotid Arteries as they rife by the fides of the Sella Turcica; and the letter (*m*) itfelf fits upon a large groove made by the Optic Nerves, where they enter into the Optic Holes.

E 2

SECOND

SECOND DIVISION.

This division shows points of the SPHOENOID also, but chiefly of the TEMPORAL BONE, and of the Corner of the PARIETAL BONE.

SPHOENOID BONE.

(*n*) Shows the Foramen Lacerum under the Wing of Ingrasias, by which all the smaller nerves enter into the socket for furnishing the eye-ball. (*o*) Shows behind that, the Foramen Rotundum for the nerve of the upper jaw : (*p*) The Foramen O-vale for the nerve of the lower jaw :—and (*q*) shows the Spinous Hole, which is large here that it may be seen, (for naturally it is extremely small), and the Groove, formed by the great artery of the Dura Mater as it enters by this spinous hole, is also seen here (*r*) marked very hard and strong.

PARIETAL BONE.

It is upon the corner of the Parietal Bone, that this groove (*r*) is formed by the artery of the Dura Mater.

TEMPORAL BONE.

The point of the Petrous Portion of the Temporal Bone is seen here projecting into the basis or floor of the cranium. The point of the triangular Petrous Portion is marked (*s*) ; and the Internal Auditory Hole, by which the auditory nerve or 7th nerve enters into the ear is marked (*t*).

THIRD DIVISION.

In this third division nothing almost but the Occipital Bone is seen ; and its parts are these.—(*u u*) The two great hollows in which the lobes of the cerebellum lie.——

2·   (*v*) (*v*) is the Ridge betwixt thefe two hollows, which rifes very high, is called the Internal Spine of the Occipital Bone, and has a fmall falx (fomewhat like the larger one) attached to it. (*w*) Marks the Foramen Lacerum, or wide irregular hole betwixt the Temporal and Occipital Bones, through which the Lateral Sinus paffes to go down into the neck, where it forms the Great Internal Jugular Vein. And the 8th pair of nerves, or Par Vagum accompanies the vein through this hole.— (*x*) Stands upon the very middle of the Cuneiform or Wedge-like Procefs of the Occipital and Sphœnoidal Bones ; for the two bones meet here, without any determined or regular limits for either.—And (*y*) ftands in the center of the Foramen Magnum, by which the Spinal Marrow goes down into the canal of the Spine.

FIGURE II.

THIS drawing explains the Bafis of the Scull, as it is turned towards the neck and throat. But this furface is fo rough, irregular, and confufed, that it will not bear that fair arrangement and complete enumeration of proceffes which the firft figure bears. The furfaces chiefly to be obferved, and, which may ferve in fome degree to arrange the fubject, are 1ft, The JAW and PALATE BONES. 2d, The Root of the TEMPORAL BONES. 3d, The LOWER PART of the OCCIPITAL BONES.

1. About the Palate we obferve,

(*a*) The Alveolar Procefs of the upper Jaw Bone, robbed of many of its teeth ; (*b*) the Palate Plate of the Upper Jaw Bone, forming a chief part of the roof of the mouth ; (*c*) the Palate Plate of the proper Palate Bone, which forms nearly one third of the Palate ; (*d*) the Tranfverfe Palate Suture, which runs acrofs the Palate, joining the Palate Bone to the Palate Procefs of the Jaw Bone ; (*e*) the Middle or Longitudinal Palate Suture, which joins the bones of the oppofite fides ; (*f*) the Foramen Incifivum, or Anterior Palatine Hole, lying juft behind the firft cutting teeth, and common to both bones ; (*g*) the pofterior Palatine Hole, which permits

the

the Palatine Nerve and Artery, to come down from the back of the noſtrils to
the Palate.

The backs of the noſtrils are formed by the riſing plates of the proper Palate Bones, and
by the Pteregoid Proceſſes. At the back of the noſtrils, we ſee, (*h*) the Vomer,
ſo named from its reſemblance to a plough-ſhare, and ſtanding exactly in the middle,
for it is the partition of the noſe; (*i*) the Outer Pteregoid Proceſs, forming the
back of the noſtrils; (*k*) the Hook of the Inner Pteregoid Proceſs, upon which the
tendon of the Tenſor Palati Muſcle turns: and a ſmall tip of the Palate Bones,
which is at this point covered by theſe Pteregoid Proceſſes of the Sphœnoid Bone, is
named, the Pteregoid Proceſs of the Palate Bone. And (*l*) marks the appearance
outwardly of the Wedge-like Proceſſes of the Occipital and Sphœnoidal Bones.

2. About the roots of the Temporal Bones we have,

(*m*) the Root of the Zygomatic Proceſs, where the Condyle of the lower Jaw plays;
and (*n*) the Ridge juſt before the Condyle, upon the top of which the Condyle ſtands,
in a dangerous ſituation, almoſt out of its ſocket when the jaws are opened wide;
and which it ſlips over, getting into the hollow for the Temporal Muſcle, when
the lower jaw is diſlocated. (*o*) Is the Mamillary, and (*p*) the Styloid Proceſs, of
the Temporal Bone. (*q*) Is the Oval Hole of the Sphœnoid Bone, for tranſmitting
the great nerve of the lower jaw. (*r*) Is the Spinous Hole of the Sphœnoid Bone,
for admitting the artery of the Dura Mater. (*s*) Is the hole near the point of the
Temporal Bone, for the Carotid Artery. (*t t t*) The Crucial Ridges of the Os Occipitis.—(*u*) The Poſterior Tuber, or the Acute and Prominent Point of the Occipital
Bone.—(*x*) The Additamentum Suturæ Lambdoidalis, which joins the back corner of the Temporal to the Occipital Bone.

The Zygoma, as formed by the Zygomatic Proceſſes of the Temporal Bone, and of
the Cheek Bone, is marked (*y*); and the hollow under the Zygoma for lodging the
Temporal Muſcle and the branch of the lower jaw to which that muſcle is attached, is marked (*z*); and is ſeen in this view on both ſides full and large.

P L A T E

SUPPLEMENTARY EXPLANATION to PLATE V. OF THE BONES.

HAVING, in doing the outline to this plate, found it poſſible to mark the points more correctly, I have added the following explanations in this ſupplementary page; and that they may unite eaſily with the firſt explanation, I repeat the eſſential points.

In the Upper Scull there are,

1. The Optic hole (*l*).

2. On each ſide of the letter (*m*), there is the likeneſs of a ſecond Optic hole, but it is merely the impreſſion which the laſt turn of the Carotid Artery makes.

3. (*n*) Is the Foramen Lacerum.

4. (*o*) Is the Foramen Rotundum.

5. (*p*) Is the Foramen Ovale.

6. (*q*) Is the Spinous Hole.

7. (*z*) Marks the round hole by which the Carotid Artery enters the ſkull, after winding through a crooked canal in the Temporal bone, about an inch in length.

8. The figure (8.) points to a great breach in the rocky part of the Temporal bone; this breach is occaſioned by the falling away of the Cartilaginous part of the Euſtachian Tube. Therefore this wide breach is found in every Church-yard ſcull; and the hole for the Carotid Artery marked (*z*), opens where this breach ends.

9. It is obſerved of the great hole marked (*w*), for the paſſage of the Jugular Vein, that it is large and irregular; that it is almoſt divided into two openings, by a ſmall projecting point; the line extending from the letter (*w*), touches exactly this ſmall point.

point. The eighth pair of nerves paſſes in the ſmaller opening before the point, the Jugular Vein paſſes in the greater opening behind it ; a ſmall bridle of the Dura Mater goes acroſs from this point, and makes the two holes diſtinct in the freſh ſcull, and defends the eighth pair of nerves from the preſſure of the Jugular Vein, when (as often happens) it is turgid with blood.

10. The number (10.) marks the hole under the Condyle by which the ninth pair of nerves, the Lingual Nerve goes out.

In FIGURE II. the chief points are theſe,

(*f*) Marks the Anterior Palatine Hole.

(*g*) Marks the Poſterior Palatine Hole.

(*h*) The Vomer, or bone forming the partition of the noſe.

(*i*) The outer Pteregoid Proceſs.

(*k*) The Inner Pteregoid Proceſs.

(*l*) The Cuneiform Proceſs of the Occipital Bone.

(1.) Marks the Foramen Lacerum, not that which is marked (*n*) in figure i. but another Foramen Lacerum belonging alſo to the orbit, not for the tranſmiſſion of nerves, but for the lodging of fat.

(*q*) Marks the Foramen Ovale.

(*r*) The Spinous Hole.

(2.) Is that great breach which is left by the fading of the Cartilaginous end of the Euſtachian Tube.

(*s*) Is the hole for the paſſage of the Carotid Artery, which as on the inſide of the ſcull opens immediately behind the breach.

(3.) Marks the great Thimble-like hole, by which the Lateral Sinus comes out from the Scull, to form the great Jugular Vein.

(4.) Is a hole ſeated behind the Condyle, the hole marked (10.) in figure i. is before the Condyle, and gives paſſage to the ninth or Lingual pair of nerves ; this ſmaller hole is behind the Condyle, and gives paſſage to a ſmall vein of the neck.

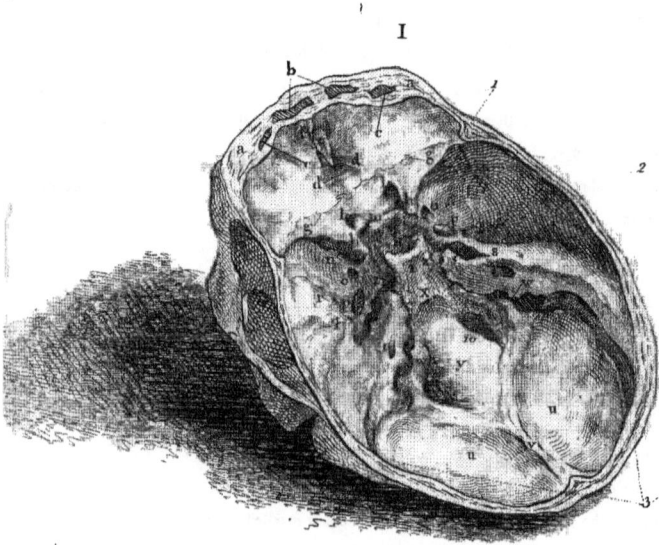

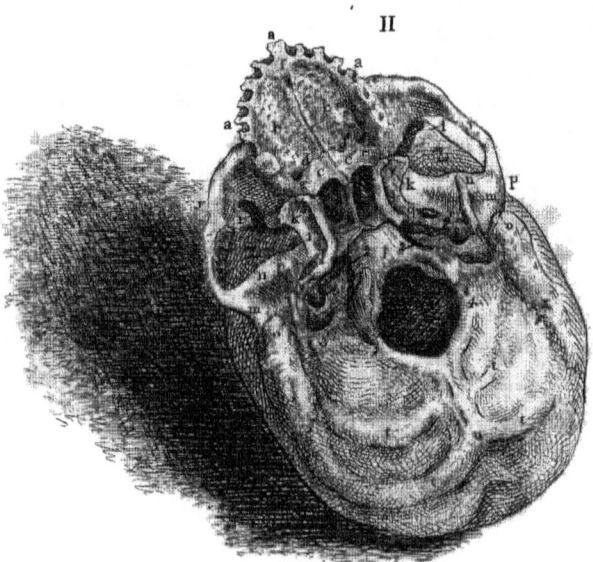

I

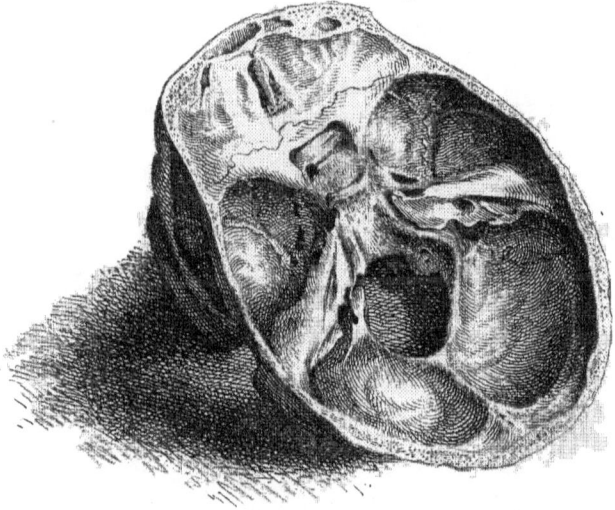

H

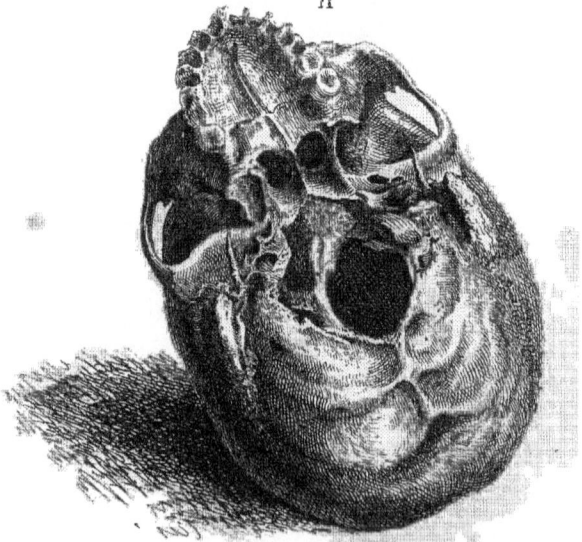

Published for the author J Bell October 1794

PLATE VI.

This Plate explains the Text Book, in all the Chapters upon the Scull.

GIVES 1*ft*, a general view of the CRANIUM, the reverfe of the firft plate; and 2*d*, a vertical fection of the Cranium, which fhews the relation and bearing of many important parts,—explains particularly the great train of finufes or cells, which make all the bafis of the Cranium hollow,—explains alfo the fpongy bones,—the Antrum Highmorianum,—the Nafal or Lachrymal Duct,—and the Mouth of the Euftachian Tube; which is feen here ftuffed out, and dried, to make its opening immediately behind the noftrils at the back of the palate more diftinct.

FIGURE I.

OUTSIDE OF THE SCULL*.

A THE Os FRONTIS; where (*a*) marks the bump of the Frontal Sinus; (*b*) The Superciliary Ridge, dotted with marks of its Nutritious Arteries; (*c*) The Superciliary Notch, and hole which the Frontal Nerve and Artery make.

B The

* Let the reader remember that there cannot be a perfect correfpondence of figures through all the plates; that no more could be attempted in the anatomy of the Bones, (a fubject fo irregular) than juft to

make

B. The Parietal Bone, and the letter is fo placed as to mark that femicircular ridge where the Temporal Mufcle arifes.

C. Marks the Temporal Bone. Where (d) marks the Meatus Auditorius; (e) the Maftoid Procefs; (f) the Zygoma; and (g) a Double Squamous Suture, as in the fcull from which this was drawn.

D. Marks the Cheek bone where all its connections are feen; (h) with the Temporal bone; (i) with the Frontal Bone; (k) with the upper Jaw Bone.

E. Marks the Wing of the Sphœnoid Bone, where it lies in the Squamous Suture; and the four corners of bone forming the Squamous Suture, are (l) the corner of the Sphœnoid (m) the corner of the Parietal; (n) the corner of the Temporal; and (o) the Corner of the Frontal Bone.

F. Marks the Small Bone of the Nofe, where the middle Nafal Suture is feen.

G. Points to the Upper Jaw Bone. The letter is placed upon the Alveolar or Socket Proceffes; and the fmall letter (p) marks the Infra Orbitary Hole.

H Marks the Lower Jaw Bone, this letter touching the point of the chin; while the fmall letter (q) marks the line of the bafis of the lower jaw; (r) the mark of the Maffeter Mufcle, the point into which it is inferted; (s) the Mental Hole by which a twig of the lower Maxillary Nerve comes out upon the face, juft as the twig of the upper Maxillary Nerve comes out upon the face by the Infra Orbitary Hole, at (p).

In the Orbit, (t) marks the holes, which being within the orbit, (for arteries and nerves paffing down into the noftril,) are called INTERNAL ORBITARY HOLES, to diftinguifh them from the Supra Orbitary and Infra Orbitary Holes. Of thefe internal Orbitary
Holes,

make each plate fyftematic and orderly in itfelf, without reference to any other plate. And fo in each plate the great letters point to the general Bone, and the leffer alphabet marks and arranges the individual parts.

Holes, one is named the ANTERIOR, the other is named the POSTERIOR, Orbitary Hole. So that in this drawing, there are seen all the holes around the Orbit, *viz.* (*r*) The Supra Orbitary Hole, or Superciliary Hole; (*p*) the Infra Orbitary Hole; and (*t*) the internal Orbitary Hole. In the orbit is seen (*u*) the Tranfverfe Suture on the right fide pure; on the left fide alfo it is feen, but appears very irregular as it really is, for it joins together a great many irregular bones.

Within the orbit fome other parts are alfo feen here, which are not fo well explained in any other plate.—The whole conftitution of the orbit is feen;—(1.) Marks the Os Unguis in its plain part, where the eye rolls upon it.——(2.) Marks the Groove of Os Unguis, where the nafal duct lies; (3.) the Os Planum, which is in fact the plain fide of the Œthmoid bone as feen Plate III. **Fig.** III. at (*e.*) (4.) Is the Orbitary Procefs of the Upper Jaw Bone. (5.) Is the Orbitary Procefs of the Sphœnoid Bone, which is exactly oppofite to its Temporal Ala or wing (E.) (6.) Is the Orbitary Plate of the Frontal Bone, which forms far the greater part of the Orbit; and (7.) at the bottom of the Orbit is the Optic hole.

In the Nofe, the letter (*v*) denotes the Vomer, the bone which forms the partition of the Nofe.

F I G U R E   II.

THE VERTICAL SECTION OF THE SCULL.

A Is the Frontal Bone; where (*a*) marks the Coronal Suture feen from within like a mere crack, and not ferrated or zig-zag, as on the outer furface of the fcull; (*b*) marks the fmall projecting Spine, to which the falx is attached, and which projects fometimes half an inch, making it impoffible to trepan fafely at this point; (*c*) the Orbitary Procefs, or plate, which lies over the eye; (*d*) the Bump mark-

F   ing

ing the Frontal Sinus or cavity. (1.) The cavity or finus itfelf, with a crofs bar in it, as there commonly is.

B The Inner Surface of the Parietal Bone; with the Artery of the Dura Mater, or rather its impreffion or furrow feen.

C The Inner Surface of the Occipital Bone; where (e) marks the Winding Groove of the Lateral Sinus; (f) that Groove ending in the thimble-like cavity, and the thimble-like cavity ending in its turn in the Foramen Lacerum, by which the finus gets out; and there paffes along with it through this wide flit, the Par Vagum, or eighth pair of nerves. (g) Marks the thicknefs of the bone, at the place of the Crucial Ridge; (h) its thinnefs, where it is loaded and preffed by the lobes of the brain. (i) Shows the fection of the Foramen Magnum. (k) Marks the Cuneiform Proceffes of the Occipital and Sphœnoidal Bones *.

D Marks the Temporal Bone, where (l) points out the Foramen Auditorium Internum, where the Auditory Nerve enters; and (m) marks the Styloid Procefs.

G Marks the Upper Jaw Bone, where it forms the Palate.

H Marks the Lower Jaw Bone, where (n) is the fection, fhowing the Cancelli of the Lower Jaw; (o) is the angle; and here upon the internal furface of the angle, the Pteregoid Mufcle is implanted; (p) the hole by which the proper nerve of the Lower Jaw, the inferior Maxillary Nerve, gets into the heart of the bone; and there going round, accompanied with an artery, a branch of each is given off to every tooth; and what remains of the Nerve and Artery after this, comes out by the Mental hole upon the chin.

The curious parts feen in this fection are;—The CELLS, SPONGY BONES, and the EUSTACHIAN TUBE.

                                                                        The

* There are two Foramina Lacera or wide holes, one belonging to the Sphœnoid Bone, in the bottom of the focket for the eye; and this one betwixt the Temporal and Occipital Bones, in the bafis of the Sull over the neck or implantation of the vertebræ.

The Cells are marked (1, 2, 3 ;) for (1.) Marks the beginning of this long train o cells, being the cells of the Frontal Bone, commonly called the Frontal Sinuses, communicating with each other, and with the nose. (2, 2, 2,) Mark the Cells of the Œthmoid Bone lying under the Cribriform Plate, and seen here by the cutting away of the Os Planum. (3.) Marks the Great Sinus of the Sphœnoid Bone. It was pretty large in this scull, and is known to belong to the Sphœnoid Bone, by the Sella Turcica and Clynoid Processes, which are seen in profile above it.

(q) Marks the back part of the Septum Nasi left; and looking past that, into the nostril, the Spongy Bones are seen ; (r) the Upper Spongy Bone is already described as a mere process of the Œthmoid Bone, hanging thus downwards into the top of the nostril : (s) the Lower Spongy Bone, is an independent separate bone ; small, as is expressed Plate IV., and hooked upon the edge of the Antrum Maxillare at this part ; the opening of the Antrum is here marked (s).

The Lachrymal Duct is marked by the probe, (t) passed upwards from the nostril, and it is seen, by the direction of this probe, that the duct opens into the nose, just under the point of the Lower Spongy Bone.

The Eustachian Tube is a large internal passage to the ear; which opens at (u) just behind the back part of the Palate, and at the back opening of the nostril : here it is well expressed, the drawing being taken from a scull which had the cartilaginous opening of the tube stuffed out and dried.

PLATE

I

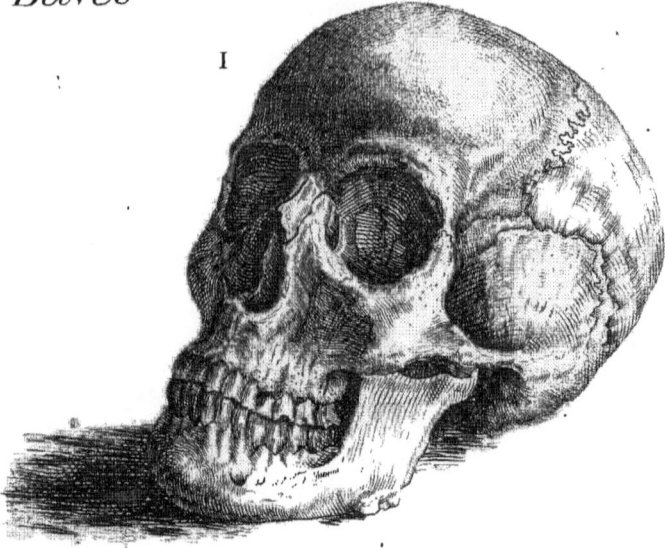

II

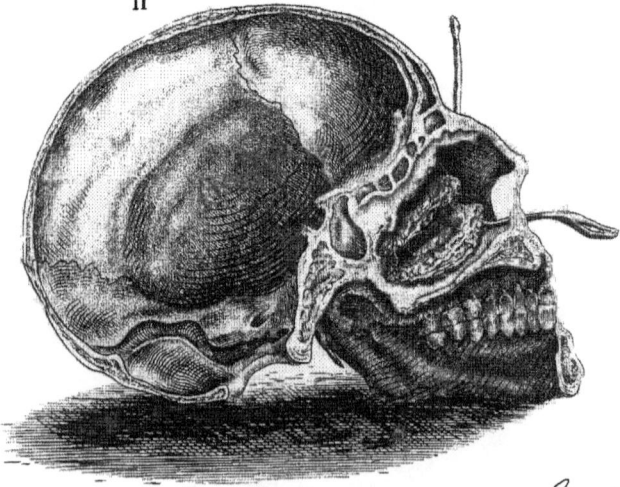

Engraved by J Bell

II

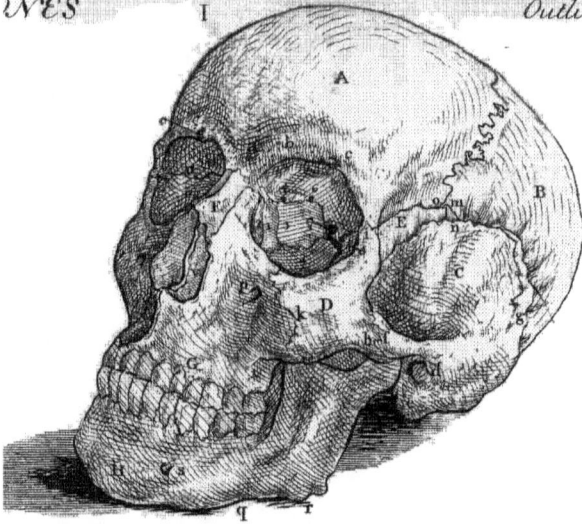

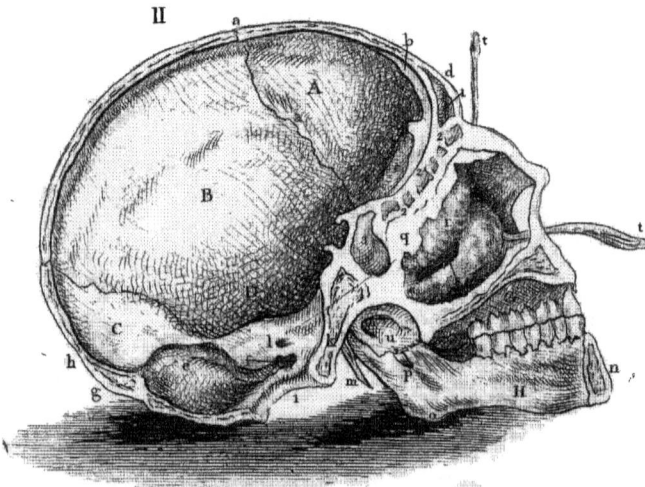

Published for the author I. Bell october 179..

Engraved by I. Bell

P L A T E   VII.

This Plate explains the Text Book, from Page 105, to Page 129.

EXPLAINS the VERTEBRÆ, with all their proceſſes and parts; and as the
ſame parts return in each Vertebra, the ſeveral Vertebræ ought to be
explained rather by ranks and orders, than as individual Bones.

FIRST ROW.

The firſt row, conſiſting of Figures I, II, and III, is drawn for the purpoſe
of contraſting the three claſſes of Vertebræ, viz. the Vertebræ of the
Back, of the Neck, and of the loins.

FIGURE   I.

REPRESENTS a Vertebra of the Loins; and the peculiarities of the Lumbar Vertebræ
are theſe.

(1.) The body is large and broad, thick, ſpongy and looſe in its texture, and tipped
with a ring, (*a*) of harder bone.

(2.) The Articulating Proceſſes, or, as they are called, the Oblique Proceſſes, are large,
for they have to bear much force; they ſtand directly upwards and downwards; the
four

four Articulating Proceſſes, (the two upper, as well as the two lower,) are marked 2, 2.

(3.) The Spinous Proceſs, is ſhort, flat, very broad, and ſtands horizontally and directly
out, ſo as not to embarraſs the motions of the loins.

(4.) The Tranſverſe Proceſs is ſhort, direct, and very ſtrong; and the Articulating
Proceſſes (2, 2) go off from the root of it.

In each Vertebra, there is formed by the roots of the Tranſverſe and Oblique Proceſſes,
where they ariſe from the body, a ring or circle of Bone, which is in each drawing
marked (*); it is for containing the Spinal Marrow.

FIGURE II.

Is a Vertebra of the Back; where,

(1.) The body is ſhorter, and is a large ſegment (viz. nearly two thirds) of a ſmall circle.

(2.) The Articulating Process is ſmall and flat, and a little inclined, but not very
oblique.

(3.) The Spinous Proceſs is long, aquiline, depreſſed to ſuch an angle that the two Spinous Proceſſes almoſt touch each other, (as is ſeen in Fig. IV.) (3. 3.) and allow of
but a very limited motion.

(4.) The Tranſverſe Proceſs is long, ſtands directly outwards, or is inclined a little upwards, and upon every dorſal vertebra there are two marks for the articulation
of the ribs; one (b) on the ſide of the vertebra itſelf, or rather betwixt the bodies of
two vertebræ, for the proper head of the rib, (Fig. X. and XI.) (1.); and again
there is another articulating ſurface (c) upon the face or fore part of the Tranſverſe
Proceſs, which is for the articulation of the little knob (Fig. X. and XI.) (3.) upon
the back part of each rib.

FIGURE

FIGURE III.

THE Cervical Vertebra has thefe chief charaters,

(1.) The body is fmall, firm, and of more folid and condenfed bone than in the vertebræ of the loins or back.

(2.) The Articulating Procefs is truely oblique.

(3.) The Spinous Procefs is fhort, and is forked.

(4.) The Tranfverfe Procefs is fhort, forked, and has a large hole in it for a great artery of the brain, which by its paffing through this canal of the vertebræ is named Vertebral Artery.

SECOND ROW.

This Row explains chiefly the conneftions of the VERTEBRÆ.

FIGURE IV.

SHows the manner in which one Dorfal Vertebra fits down upon another, fo that the Articulating Proceffes (2, 2.) check upon one another, and the Spinous Proceffes (3, 3) are feen to be long and aquiline, and lying fo over each other as to prevent all motion backwards or forwards, while the ribs limit the motion to either fide. But in this drawing the one Spinous Procefs is tilted up from the other a little, owing to the want of that intervertebral fubftance which fhould lie betwixt the bodies. The hole is feen here at (d) betwixt the two vertebræ, by which a nerve goes off at the interftice between each Vertebra: fo there are in all twenty-four nerves of the Spine, correfponding with the number of Vertebræ in the Spine.

FIGURE

FIGURE V.

T WO Dorsal Vertebræ are here seen in their right position, connected by the intervertebral substance; with the end of one rib in its place; and at (*b*) is seen one articulating surface on the body of the vertebra naked. At (*c*) is seen the articulating
surface, upon the face of the Transverse Procefs, naked. At (*d*) is seen the head of
the rib covering the two articulating surfaces; connected at (*e*) with the body, and
at (*f*) with the Transverse Procefs of its own vertebra.

FIGURE VI.

I S a drawing of the INTERVERTEBRAL SUBSTANCE, which is of that ambiguous nature,
that anatomists chooſe this name, to avoid the dilemma of calling it either Cartilage or
Ligament, when it has not the character diſtinctly either of Cartilage or of Ligament.
It is ſhown here as it is found betwixt the Lumbar Vertebræ; and the concentric
circles of which it conſiſts are better expreſſed towards the margin (*g*); but towards
the centre, and eſpecially in the very middle, it becomes ſoft, pulpy, the circles confuſed. The ſubſtance is ſo much ſofter in the centre, that there is almoſt a hole at (*b*);
eſpecially when the bone is allowed to ſpoil a little, as this one was. At (*i*) is
ſeen a ſlight indication of the Spinal marrow, (which was alſo corrupted,) going down
through the great hole of the vertebra.

THE THIRD ROW.

Explains the forms of the ATLAS and DENTATUS; the two Vertebræ by which almoſt
all the motions of the head are performed. Fig. VII. explains the Atlas;
Fig. VIII. explains the Dentatus; Fig. IX, ſhows the way in which the Atlas fits
down upon the tooth-like procefs and oblique ſhoulders of the Dentatus.

FIGURE

FIGURE VII.

EXPLAINS the Atlas, or first Vertebra, where we find,

(1.) The body entirely wanting, and the place of the body supplied by Articulating Surfaces (2, 2), so large as to give sufficient strength and thickness to the sides of the ring.

N. B. At the place where the body should be, there is at (*k*) a smooth Articulating Surface for the Tooth-like Procefs of the Atlas rolling. There is at (*l*) a little tip or point, which is tied by ligaments to the margin of the Occipital Hole; at (*m*) there is a fort of straitening in the ring, and at this point a ligament goes acrofs the ring, dividing it into two, and holding firm the tooth-like procefs.

(2.) The Oblique or Articulating Procefles of this vertebra are oval, and of a converging form; and this peculiarity in their direction limits the motions of the head, so that it cannot turn, but only nod, upon the Atlas.

(3.) The Spinous Procefs is wanting. A fmall knob reprefents the fpinous procefs; and the want of this fpine enables the Atlas to turn freely in circles upon the Dentatus.

(4.) The Tranfverfe Procefs, alfo ending in a little knob, and perforated by the large hole for the Vertebral Artery.

FIGURE VIII.

THE DENTATUS, where the points of defcription are,

(1.) The whole body of the Vertebra, rifing gradually towards the apex or point of its axis or tooth-like procefs, which is marked (*m*).

(2.) The broad flat articulating furfaces, like fhoulders, at the root of the tooth-like procefs; upon which the atlas refts and turns.

G

3. The

(3.) The Spinous Procefs is fhort, thick, and forked.

(4.) The Tranfverfe Procefs fhort, knobby, and perforated with the Vertebral Hole.

(*n*) Marks the Neck or Collar, the narrow part of the Tooth-like Procefs, where it is embraced by the Atlas ;——and (*m*) marks the Apex or pointed extremity of the Tooth-like Procefs.——(*o*) Shows how deep the ring of this particular vertebra is, and how fairly triangular its great hole for the paffage of the fpinal marrow is.

F I G U R E   IX.

Explains the manner of connection betwixt the ATLAS and the DENTATUS ; fhows the ring of the Atlas fet down upon the fhoulders of the Dentatus ;——and here all the parts are marked with the fame numbers as in the other drawings.

F I G U R E   X. AND XI.

Are DRAWINGS OF THE RIBS : where we fee,—(1.) the Head of the Rib, by which it is joined to the body of the vertebra.——(2.) The Neck or ftraitning beyond the head.—(3.) The Tubercle by which it is articulated with the Tranfverfe Procefs.—— (4.) Another little Tubercle, beyond this fecond articulating furface.——(5.) The Angle of the Rib, or the point from which it begins to bend forwards, (*p*) the Groove in which the intercoftal artery lies. (*q*) The more fpongy end of the rib, with a fort of rude focket, which receives the cartilage that joins it to the fternum.

F I G U R E   XII.

Represents the WHOLE LENGTH of the STERNUM.

(1.) Marks the Upper Part of the Sternum ; where (*r*) fhows the pointed part of this

firft

firſt bone turned downwards to meet the ſecond piece of the Sternum. (*s*) Is a hollow which makes way for the Trachea, &c. (*t t*) Are two articulating ſurfaces, by which the clavicle of either ſide is joined to this piece of the ſternum.

(2.) The ſecond piece of the Sternum, of great length, receiving the cartilages of moſt of the ribs; and the ſockets for receiving the cartilages are ſeen, though not very fully all along its edge at (*u u*) &c.

(3.) Is the Enſiform Cartilage, which in moſt bodies is ſtraight pointed, as in this drawing, but ſometimes bifurcated;—ſometimes bent down, or on the contrary turned remarkably upwards; very ſeldom oſſified, except in thoſe perſons who are extremely old.

G 2

PLATE

I

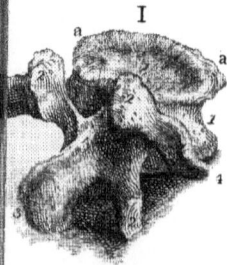

III

II

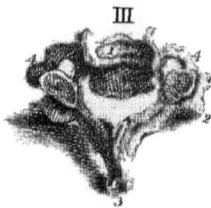

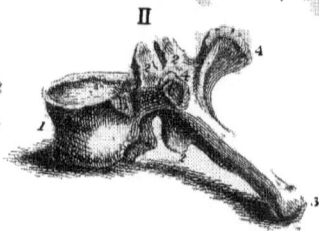

V

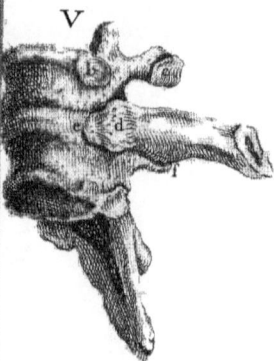

VI

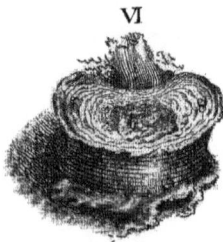

IV

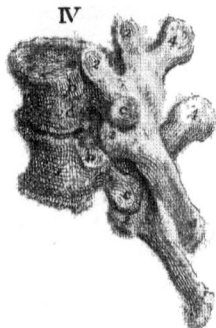

VII

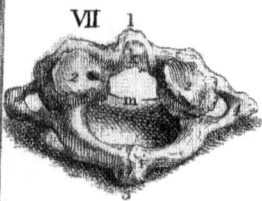

IX

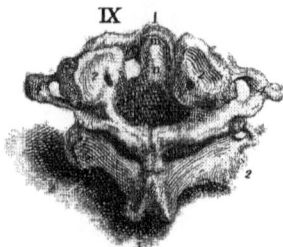

VIII

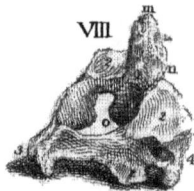

XII

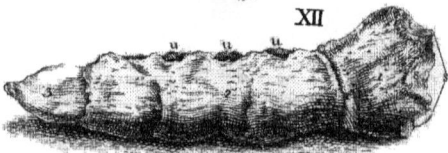

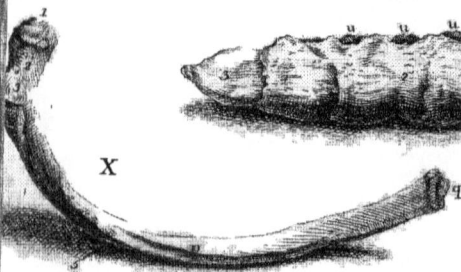

X

XI

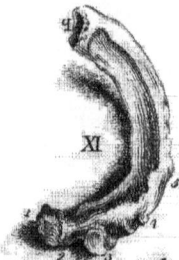

Published for the auth. L.Wall october 1799

Etched by Bell

PLATE VIII.

This Plate explains the Text Book, from Page 105, to Page 147.

Is a general view of all the BONES OF THE TRUNK. It is chiefly ufeful by fhowing the general pofition of Bones which have been already minutely explained, and requires only a very loofe and general explanation, becaufe it is a general plate merely, upon which the parts and proceffes need not be minutely told.

A The Ring of the firft Vertebra or Atlas.

B The Tip of the Tooth-like Proceffes of the Dentatus.

C The Bodies of the Cervical Vertebræ.

D Their Tranfverfe Proceffes.

E The Holes betwixt the Vertebræ, by which the Cervical Nerves come out from the canal of the fpinal marrow.

F The Firft Rib, lying flat and level here ; and it is at this place, betwixt the clavicle and the firft rib that the fubclavian veffels come out.

G The General Convex of the Thorax, formed by the middle of the ribs.—(*a a a*) Mark the ends of the ribs which receive the cartilages, by which the ribs are joined to the fternum.

G Marks the Seven True Ribs.

H

H Marks the 3 firft Falfe Ribs, whofe cartilages run into the cartilage of the feventh rib.

I Marks the Two Loofe or floating Ribs, whofe cartilages do not join the other cartilages, nor are united to the fternum ; but ftand out in the flanks, free and independent, their cartilages being buried in the thick flefh of the abdominal mufcles.

K The Cartilages of the Ribs.

L The Firft or triangular piece of the Sternum.

M The Second or long piece, which receives almoft all the Cartilages.

N The Third peice, as it is ufually called ; though it is merely Cartilage, to extreme old age.—This 3d piece N is the Cartilago Mucronata, Enfiformis, or Swordlike.

O The Clavicle, or Collar Bone, as it lies upon the top of the cheft ; and here it is feen how the bone by its proper pofition, keeps off and fupports the fcapula or fhoulder-blades.

P Marks the lower border of the Scapula. (b) Marks the Acromian Procefs, to which the Clavicle is connefted.—(c) is the Glenoid or Articulating Cavity, for holding the fhoulder bone ; (d) is the Caracoid Procefs, fhowing how it projects on the infide of the joint, in the hollow under the arch of the Clavicle.—It is plain from this pofition of the procefs, that it fhould be felt on the breaft juft above the border of the Axilla.

Q The bodies of the Lumbar Vertebræ, thick and maffy to fupport the weight of all the parts above.

R The Tranfverfe Proceffes of the Lumbar Vertebræ, (a a) touch the Spinous Proceffes, where they appear in the interftices of the Tranfverfe ones.——(e e e) Mark the intervertebral fubftances, or rather reprefent the putty, which is put betwixt the Vertebræ (in making our fkeleton) to ftand, in place of the interverte-bral fubftance.

S The Os Sacrum ; where (f f) reprefent the holes of the Sacrum difpofed regular-ly in pairs.—(g g) Reprefent the white lines, which were cartilaginous in the child dividing the Sacrum into five pieces, but are now confolidated into white lines of pro-minent bone particularly hard and firm. —— (h) Reprefents the joining of the Sacrum to the Os Ilium at either fide, which joining is named the Sacro-Iliac Symphyfis.

T That

T That divifion of the Os Innominatum, which is called the Os Ilium; where (*i*) marks the hollow bofom of that expanded wing, which lying obliquely outwards like the wing of a chariot, is called the Ala Ilii: the Iliacus Internus Mufcle, arifes from this furface. — (*k*) Is the circle called the Spine or Ridge of the Os Ilium.—-(*l*) Is the fudden fharp point, by which the Spine ends, and which is there named the Spinous Procefs, to which the name Anterior is added, to diftinguifh it from others, which lie concealed in the joining with the Sacrum. This Anterior Superior Spinous Procefs has another under it fmaller and marked (*m*), which is called the Anterior Inferior Spinous Procefs.——It is merely a fmall Bump, over the top of the focket for the origin of the Rectus Mufcle. (*n*) Marks the back or Dorfum Ilii, from which the Glutæi Mufcles arife.

U U Thefe two letters interfect all that part of the Os Innominatum, which is called Ifchium; where (*o*) marks the body of the bone, where it forms a chief fhare in the focket. (*p*) Marks the Spinous Procefs, which is feen through the opening of the Pelvis projecting towards the Sacrum.——(*q*) Marks the Tuberofity or Bump of the Os Ifchium, the loweft point of the Pelvis, and the part upon which we reft in fitting; and (*r*) marks the Ramus, or branch of the *Ifchium*, as it rifes to meet a like branch of the Pubis.

V Marks the third piece of the Os Innominatum, *viz.* the Pubis;—where (*s*) is the body, where it forms part of the focket for the thigh-bone; —— (*t*) the higheft point named Crifta Pubis;——(*u*) points to the Symphifis Pubis, or joining of the oppofite bones;—(*v*) marks the leg of the Pubis, defcending to meet the leg of the Ifchium. The Rami of the Ifchium and of the Pubis form, with the other parts of the Os Innominatum; firft the Arch of the Pubis;—fecondly, the Thyroid Hole; and the Rami are faid to meet one half belonging to the Pubis, and one half to the Ifchium, becaufe they are in fact feparate in the child; a clear tranfparent cartilage, being interpofed betwixt them.——(*x*) Marks this Thyroid Hole; and (*y*) marks the Acetabulum or focket for the thigh bone.

P L A T E

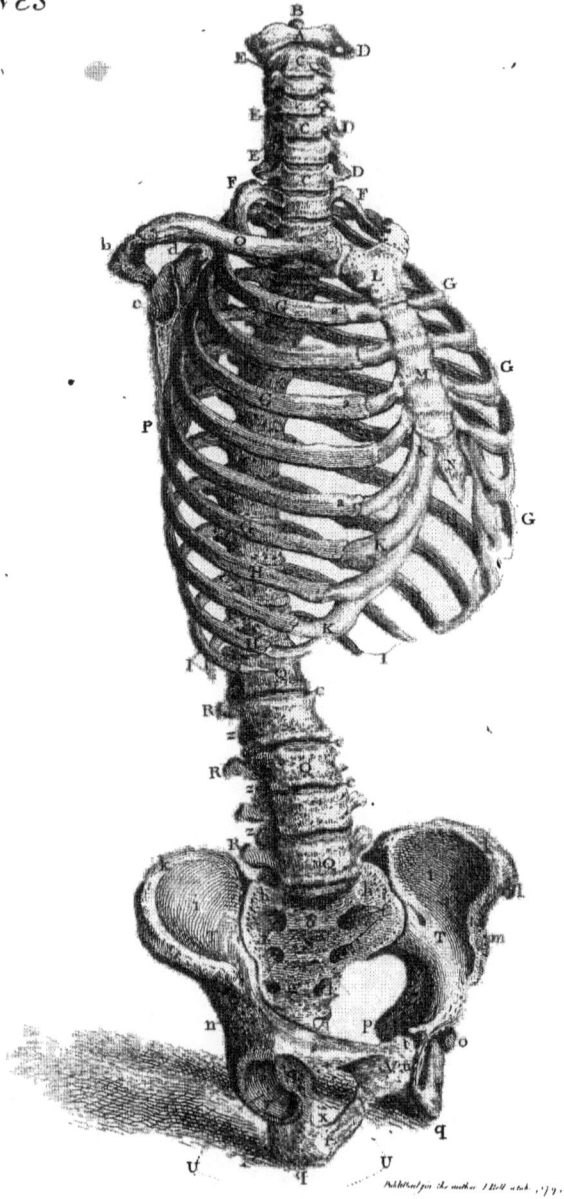

Publish'd as the author J Bell et tab. '79.

P L A T E   IX.

This Plate explains the Text Book, from Page 147, *to Page* 158.

REPRESENTS the THIGH BONE, TIBIA, and FIBULA.

F I G U R E S   I. AND II.

REPRESENT the fore and back views of the THIGH BONE.——And in order that the
letter prefs may proceed in the regular order of a little defcription or demonftration,
the fmall figures are put upon each drawing; fo that any number that is wanting on
one drawing, muft be found on the other.

The FIRST FIGURE fhows the Back Part of the Thigh Bone, which is marked by our feeing
here, from behind, the length of the neck of the bone ;—the manner of its rifing out
of the two great proceffes, the Trochanters ;—the projection and roughnefs of the
Linea Afpera, and the deep hollow betwixt the Condyles.

The SECOND FIGURE, or the fore view, is exceedingly fimple, having no ftrong marks.
The Linea Afpera is turned almoft out of fight. The chief peculiarity of the fore
view is, that it fhows the bending form of the bone.

H

THE

THE POINTS OF DESCRIPTION ARE,

(1.) The Body :———very thick, ſtrong, of a cylindrical form, bending outwards with a gentle curve.

(2.) The Head, which is very ſmooth, and very fairly circular. It is a large ſegment of a ſmall circle, and is let pretty deep down into its ſocket. There is a dimple at *(a)*, which marks the place where the central ligament once was.

(3.) The Neck of the Bone, long, and almoſt horizontal, to ſet the ſhaft of the bone the wider off from the Haunch Bone, that it may move freely.

(4.) The great Trochanter, a large bump or proceſs for the inſertion of the Glutæi Muſcles.

(5.) The leſſer Trochanter, a ſmaller proceſs, for the inſertion of many muſcles which move the Thigh Bone inwards.

(6.) The Linea Aſpera, or rough line, from which much of the Muſcular fleſh that covers the thigh ariſes.———And this Linea Aſpera, or rough line begins at *(b)* in a forking form from the roots of each Trochanter :———the two lines meet, and the Linea Aſpera becomes ſingle in the middle of the thigh, *(c)*—Towards its lower end *(d)* it forks again to go off towards each Condyle.

(7.) The two Condyles, which form the great articulating ſurfaces of the Thigh Bone, where it lies in the knee-joint.—In Fig. II. we ſee that the inner Condyle *(e)* is the larger one ; being larger to compenſate for the oblique direction of the thigh bone. At *(f)* Fig. II. we ſee, covered with cartilage, the flat poliſhed ſurface upon which the Rotula or knee-pan rolls.—And in Fig. I. at *(g)* we ſee the very deep notch betwixt the two Condyles, in which the crucial ligaments of the knee-joint lie.

FIGURE

FIGURE III.

THE TIBIA.

THIS is a drawing of the right TIBIA, feen from before. The upper end belonging
to the knee is large and broad, and is likened to the trumpet end of a pipe.——The
lower head belonging to the ancle is fmall, and has one projecting point, *viz.* that
which forms the inner ancle, and which is thought to refemble the flute-mouth of a
pipe. The whole Bone has the triangular or prifmatic form of the Ulna and Radius.

(1.) Is the Upper head of the Tibia belonging to the knee joint ; where *(b)* marks a little tubercle or rifing, which divides the two articulating furfaces from each other. It is
from the back part of this tubercle, that the crofs ligaments of the knee joint arife.
(i i) Mark the two lunar hollows, upon which the two Condyles of the thigh bone
reft, and in which the femilunar or moveable cartilages of the knee joint lie. *(k)* Is
that rough circle which bounds the articulating furface, and from which the Capfular
Ligament arifes. *(l)* Is the tubercle or bump of the Tibia, upon which we reft in
kneeling, and into which the great fore tendon called the Ligament of the Patella is
fixed : and *(m)* is the prominent ridge of the fhin, which begins from this tubercle,
and goes downwards in the waving form of an Italic *f*. *(u)* Is that part of the Tibia
which receives the upper end of the Fibula.

(2.) Is the middle part of the Bone, which is of a triangular or prifmatic form, and the
figure (2) is repeated upon each of the three angles.

(3.) Is the lower and fmaller head of the Bone belonging to the ancle joint ; where *(n)*
marks the fmooth hollow which receives the bones of the foot, and which is named
(like the articulating furface of the Radius), the Scaphoid, or Boat-like Cavity of the
Tibia. *(o)* Marks the projection or procefs of the inner ancle, which guards the
joint, preventing luxation inwards. *(p)* Is the fmall cavity on the fide of the
Tibia, which receives the lower head of the Fibula, in the way that is reprefented
in next plate.

H 2   FIGURE

FIGURE   IV.

I S a drawing of the Fibula, which is a long flender bone, fo extremely fimple in its
form, that there needs be no further defcription than this, that the fhaft of the bone
(q) is exceedingly flender,——is much longer than the Tibia,—and is triangular like
the Tibia. The upper end (r) is laid under the projecting head of the Tibia, at (u
Fig. III.) and it is laid flat upon it; fo that this articulating and fmooth furface (r)
is fmooth only for the fake of a very flight degree of fhuffling motion.

The lower end (s) is the larger.—It unites with the lower end of the Tibia (p Fig. III.)
to form the ancle joint. This guards the ancle joint without, as the Procefs of the
Tibia guards it within. And this fmooth articulating furface (t) is for receiving the
fide of the Aftragalus, that bone of the foot by which chiefly the ancle joint is formed.

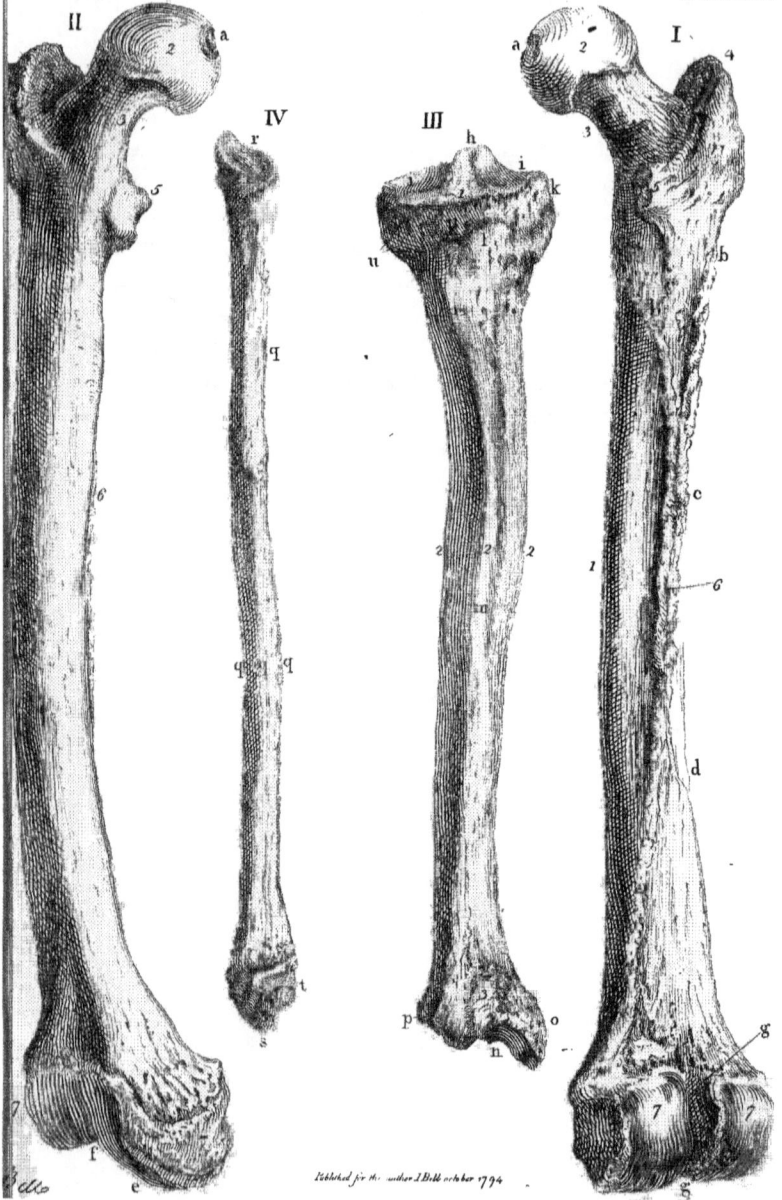

II a 2 3 5 6 7 e f

IV r q q q t s

III h i k u 2 2 2 n p n o

I a 2 4 3 b c 6 1 d g 7 7 g

Published for the author J. Bell october 1794

PLATE X.

This Plate explains the Text Book, from Page 153, to Page 166.

EXPLAINS the CONNECTIONS of the TIBIA and FIBULA, and all the BONES of the FOOT and of the TOES.

FIGURE I.

SHOWS the TIBIA and FIBULA laid to each other as they lie in the leg; and here all the letters and figures, explaining the Tibia and Fibula of the laſt plate are put upon the very ſame points; ſo that no new letters nor figures are required, except (*v*), to mark that ſpace betwixt the Tibia and Fibula in which the Inter-oſſeous Membrane lies; and (*x*) to ſhow the arch which is made by (*o*) the procefs of the inner ancle, and (*s*) the lower head of the Fibula forming the outer ancle: for the deepneſs of the arch, and the projection of theſe two points, ſhow how very ſecure the ancle joint is; the ſmooth head of the Aſtragalus marked (*a* Pl. X. Fig. IV.) being received deep into this arch.

FIGURE

FIGURE II.

SHows the Outer Surface of the Rotula or Patella, which is rough, and marked with many points where its nutritious arteries enter.

FIGURE III.

SHows the Lower Surface of the Patella, viz. that which is turned towards the cavity of the joint; and here there is seen a rising line at (*,) which lies in the great hollow betwixt the two Condyles;—while the two hollows on each side of this rising move upon the convexities of the Condyles. In short, this smooth inner surface of the patella is moulded as it were upon the surface marked (f) in the last plate, Figure II.

FIGURE IV. and V.

EXPLAIN all the Bones of the Foot, viz. of the TARSUS or instep, of the METATARSUS, and of the TOES.

The bones of the Tarsus are 7 in number, fewer and larger than the bones of the Carpus.

(1.) The Astragalus is that great bone which immediately forms the ancle joint;—where (a) marks the great ball or cartilaginous pully which is received into the arch formed by the Tibia and Fibula.——(b) Is the flat side of the bone upon which the processes of the inner and outer ancles lie, embracing the joint closely.—— (c) Is a little flat neck or projection which lies over the heel-bone. (d) Is the neck of that large round head which makes a ball and socket joint with the Os Naviculare, which is marked (3).

(2.)

(2.) The Os Calcis lies under the Aftragalus, and is the largeft of the Tarfal Bones, fupporting all the weight of the body; and here thefe points chiefly are feen.—(*e*) The tip of the bone, which looks upwards, receiving the Tendo Achillis, or great Back Tendon. —— (*f*) The loweft rough point ; the point of the heel upon which we ftand.—— (*g*) The head, by which the Os Calcis is joined to the Os Cuboides, marked (7.) the Os Cuboides being received at this part into a large hollow focket of the Os Calcis.

(3.) Is the Os Naviculare or Scaphoides, whichhas been fo named from its refemblance to a boat. But if there be any fuch refemblance it is effectually concealed in all thefe views. The Os Naviculare has rifing edges and a fair round focket, which is turned towards the Aftragulus (1.) to receive the large round head of that bone.

(4, 5, and 6.) Are the Cuneiform or Wedge-like Bones ; and in this view the fquare external furfaces chiefly are feen ;—and thefe Cuneiform Bones, ought juft to be reckoned fimply according to their order, the firft, fecond, and third cuneiform bones, beginning with that which fupports the great toe.

(7.) The Os Cuboides is a large fquare or cube like bone, as its name implies, but by no means a regular cube.——It forms a large fhare of the Tarfus, and fupports the Metatarfal Bone of the Little Toe.

The Cuneiform Bones are lefs eafily underftood, and I have therefore made a fecond drawing of the foot, Fig. V. (where the fame letters and marks are ftill preferved,) in which I have fhown the point of the Cuneiform Bones, the Metatarfal ones being taken away. In this figure the faces of the Cuboid and of the Cuneiform Bones are directly feen. And it is underftood why they are called Cuneiform or wedge-like bones, for the upper furfaces marked (4, 5, 6,) are broad and fquare ; —— while their lower furfaces at (*) are fmall and pointed ; Thefe fmaller ends of the wedges being turned inwards or towards the foal of the foot. In Fig. IV. (*b*) marks the five Metatarfal Bones ; fo named from their being placed on

the

the Tarfus.—(i) Marks the firft rank or phalanx,—(k) the fecond,—(l) the third rank
of the bones of the toes.

FIGURE VI.

SHows the foot in profile, and explains particularly well the large head of the Aftragalus (d). Thefe drawings are juft half the fize of nature, whence it may eafily be underftood how large this head of the aftragalus is ;—as large fully as the head of the
fhoulder bone ;—and the focket of the Os Naviculare, (3), into which this head of
the aftragalus is received, is both larger and a deeper circle than the Glenoid Cavity
of the Scapula, into which the head of the fhoulder bone is received.

The manner in which the procefs (c) of the Aftragalus is joined with the Os Calcis, (2) fo
as to allow of a fhuffling motion, is alfo explained here.   The great length of the firft
bone, or Metatarfal Bone of the great toe (b) is alfo to be obferved, becaufe it is fometimes to be cut away ; and it fhould not be forgotten that it goes very deep into the foot.

The fmall bone, commonly called Sefamoid Bone, from its refembling, or being thought
to refemble, a grain of Sefamum (though it is much larger), is feen here at (m) lying
under the ball of the great toe, where it is connected with the tendons of the fhort
flexor mufcles of the great toe.——There are commonly two under the ball of
each great toe, and there are occafional Sefamoid bones under the other toes, and
fometimes under the great joint of the thumb.

The feveral Phalanges, as they are called, or ranks of bones in the toes, need not a-
gain be explained.

The only important point remaining to be explained, is the double arch of the foot ; for
there are two arches. Firft (n) the great and general arch ;——the two points of
which are the tip of the heel, and the ball of the great toe. Thefe points alone of all
the foot touch the ground.—The elafticity of this arch, proceeding from its numerous bones and their joinings, gives a fpring and eafe in the ftep ; and the arch

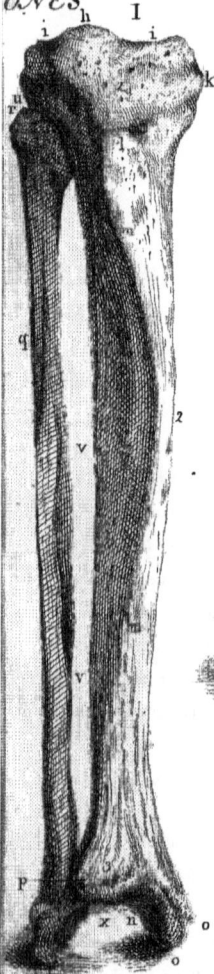

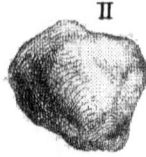

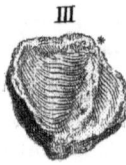

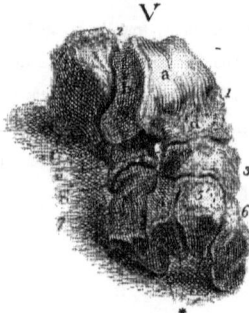

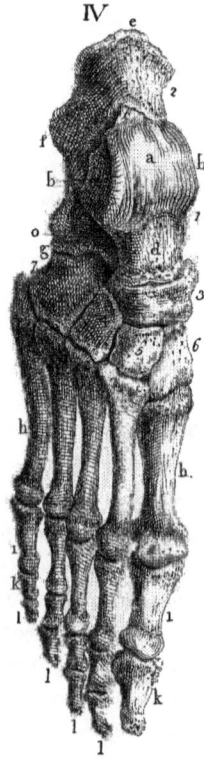

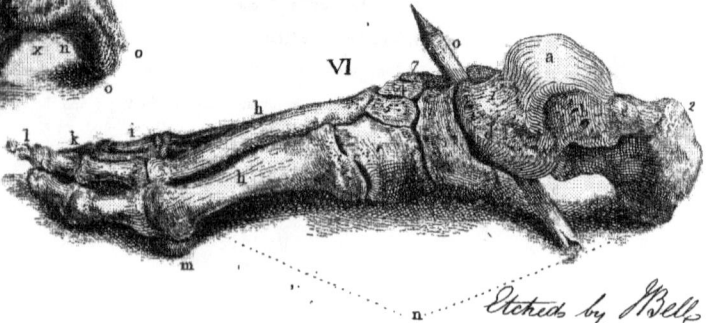

I

II

III

IV

V

VI

Etched by I Bell

Publ. May 1. Bell fec. 1794

is fupported under the weight of the whole body, both by the particular ligaments belonging to the individual joints of the foot,—and more particularly by the Great Fafcia or ligament, (I would call it,) of the fole of the foot, which from one point (the heel) extends to the root of each toe individually.

But there is alfo a fecond and particular arch, which the bones of the Tarfus form among themfelves. This arch is explained by fhowing a large central hole, which is ex-preffed in each of thefe drawings, and is marked (o).—In Fig. IV. there is only a darknefs fhowing where this central hole is.—In Fig. V. the hole is feen fair (by the Tarfus being turned round, and is marked (o). In Fig. VI. it is explained by a broken pencil, (o) thruft up through this central opening.

I   P L A T E

P L A T E   XI.

This Plate explains the Text Book, from Page 166, to Page 177.

OF the SCAPULA, CLAVICLE, and ARM BONE.

F I G U R E S I. AND II.

EXPLAIN the Scapula, fhowing, 1*ft*, its internal,—2*dly*, its external furface.

The Scapula or Shoulder Blade, is of a triangular fhape. (*a*) Marks its flat furface, which is turned towards the ribs, hollow, to fuit the convexity of the ribs.——And the letter (*a*) is repeated all over the furface, to fhow the little rifings of this furface; for this is the part upon which the Sub-fcapular Mufcle lies; and thefe rifings are the marks of its fibres.

(*b*) Shows the Outer Surface of the Scapula, which is in its turn a little convex;—is croffed by the Spine, or that high ridge (8) which divides it into two furfaces;—the lower furface (*c*) holding the infra-fpinatus;—the upper furface (*d*) holding the fupra-fpinatus mufcle.

THE LINES AND PROCESS OF THE SCAPULA ARE THESE;

(1.) Is the upper Cofta or border of the Scapula, where (*e*) marks a notch, which is fometimes a complete hole, or when incomplete it is made out by a ligament. It gives paffage to the Scapular arteries and nerves.

I 2

(2.) The

(2.) Is the Lower Cofta or border, which is round, and at the place (*f*) gives origin to the Teres Major and Teres Minor mufcles.

(3.) This long fide is called the Bafis of the Scapula, and has the great Trapezoid and Rhomboid Mufcles implanted into it from above and behind; while the Serratus Anticus is implanted into it from before and from below.

(4.) Shows the Upper Angle which receives the Levator Scapulæ Mufcle.

(5.) The Lower Angle.

(6.) The Glenoid or Articulating Cavity, which is particularly fmall and fuperficial, confidering how large the head of the fhoulder bone is.

(7.) The Neck of the Scapula fo called; it is the fmaller part which fupports the head, though, properly fpeaking, there is no neck;—and when the head of the fhoulder bone is faid, in a luxation, to lie upon the neck of the Scapula, it lies upon the place marked (*g*).

(8.) The Spine of the Scapula, which divides the upper furface, and which, rifing higher as it goes forwards, terminates at laft in the Acromion Procefs.

(9.) Is the Acromion Procefs; it is juft the end of the fpine, which turns its flat fide towards the head of the fhoulder bone, and overhangs the fhoulder to defend the joint, and prevent luxations upwards.

(10.) And there is ftill a farther fecurity; for the Coracoid Procefs (10) ftands upon the inner fide of the joint, and defends it within. It is named Coracoid Procefs, from its being crooked like the beak of a crow.

FIGURE III.

Explains the Clavicle or Collar Bone: a bone which is extremely fimple in its form, and has few or no parts;—and in which the letter (*h*) marks the middle, the roundeft part of the bone, that point which is moft prominent in the breaft; the part moft frequently broken. (*i*) Marks the end neareft the Thorax, and fhows

the

the circular articulating furface, by which it is joined to the Sternum ; and under this end a fmall moveable cartilage lies. (*k*) Marks the outer end, or that which is turned towards the fhoulder blade : the Clavicle is flattened at this end, and touches the Acromion by one fingle point only.

FIGURE IV.

THE Os Humeri, Shoulder Bone, or Arm Bone.

(1.) The head is large,—flat,—is a fmall fegment of a large circle,—feems quite dif-proportioned to its focket, (6. Fig. I. II.)

(2.) Is the neck as it is called; though there is no proper neck ; there being no length, nor narrower part betwixt the body and the head of the bone.

(3.) The Greater Tuberofity.

(4.) The Leffer Tuberofity ;—the Greater and Leffer Tuberofities being two knobs, for the infertion of thofe mufcles which come from the Scapula.

(5.) Is the Groove betwixt thefe tuberofities, for the paffage of the long tendon of the Biceps Mufcle, which runs here as a rope does in its pulley.

(*a*) Marks the roughnefs about one third down the arm bone, into which the tendon of the Deltoides is implanted.

(*b*) Marks the place, where (a little below its middle) the Os Humeri turns flatter, be-caufe it is to terminate flat and broad, to favour the hinge-like joining of the bones of the fore arm ; and

(6.) Shows one ridge on the inner fide of the arm bone ;

(7.) Shows another fimilar ridge or edge of the bone, on its inner fide—each ridge run-ning down towards its own Condyle.

(8.) Is the external Condyle, fmaller and lefs projecting, becaufe it gives origin only to the extenfors of the hand and fingers, a fet of mufcles which do not need much power nor the advantage of a long lever.

(9.) Is

(9.) Is the inner Condyle, which is very long and very prominent, to give a greater
power to thofe mufcles which bend the hand and fingers.

The elbow joint, being a very ftrict and limited hinge, has a long articulating furface :—
and there are properly two furfaces, one for the Radius, and one for the Ulna.

(10.) Is the longer articulating furface, to which the Ulna is fo joined as to perform none
but hinge-like motions.

(11.) Is a neat fmall round knob, tipped with fmooth articular cartilage ; and to this
fmall knob, the face of the button-like end of the radius is applied ; and by the
roundnefs of this knob the radius is enabled to perform not only the hinge-like
motions to accompany the motion of the Radius ; but alfo its own free circular
motions, by which the hand is carried round.

(12.) Is that very deep hole which the Coronoid Procefs of the ulna checks into.

(13.) There is a fimilar one marked (13,) which belongs to the demonftration of the fore
part of the fhoulder-bone, and is to be feen by turning to the next plate.

IV

I

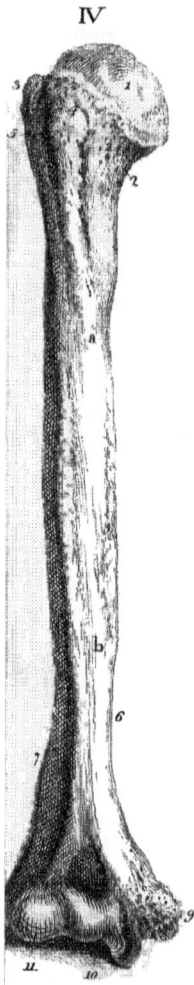

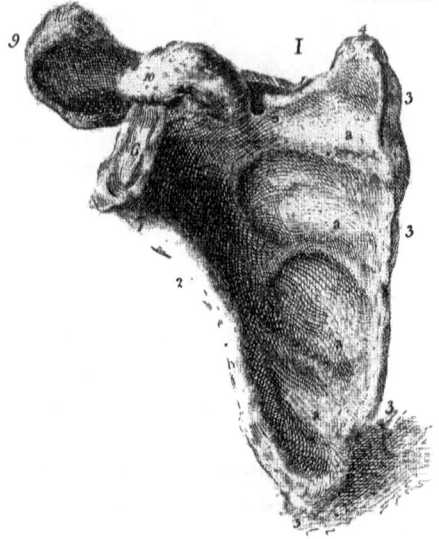

II

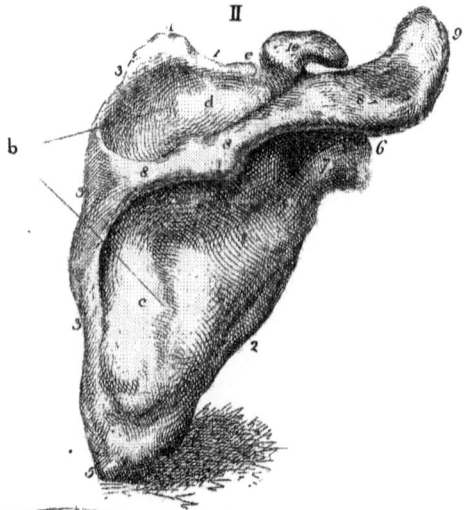

III

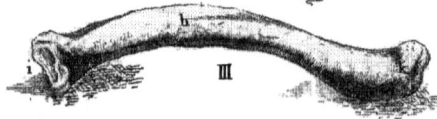

Published for the work, J.B. October 1794

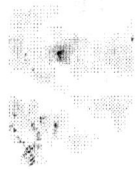

PLATE XII.

This Plate explains the Text Book, from Page 177, to Page 190.

Explains the Radius and Ulna, Carpus and Fingers.

FIGURE I.

In the drawing of the Os Humeri, all the defcriptions and letters belonging to the laft plate belong equally to this. This drawing were fuperfluous, but for the important purpofe of fhowing the back part of the articulating furface, where we do not find that round furface marked (11) in the laft plate, and which is called the Leffer Head of the Humerus, but only the hinge-like furface for the articulation of the Ulna. And the chief object of this drawing, is to fhow, that here alfo upon the back part of the bone, there is a deep hollow betwixt the Condyles ; on the fore part of the bone the hollow is for receiving the Coronoid Procefs of the Ulna, which checks into that hollow when the arm is bent forwards; but here upon the back part, this deep hollow, marked (13,) receives the Olecranon, or great procefs of the Ulna, when the arm is extended. It is alfo to be obferved; that in this drawing the twifted form of the bone is well expreffed and truely, not caricatured ; for the edge does in fact turn thus round.

2   FIGURE

FIGURE II.

THE ULNA.

THE Ulna is the longer of the two bones which lie in the fore arm. The whole bone is of a triangular shape, with 3 sharp edges; the upper end is larger, and belongs to the elbow joint; the lower or Little Head belongs to the wrist. The bone has these points of description.

(1.) Is the great cavity, which receives the lower end of the *humerus* to form the elbow joint, and this is called the Greater Sigmoid cavity.

(2.) The Olecranon, a large tubercle which marks the point of the elbow upon which we rest, and guards the Sigmoid Cavity behind.

(3.) The Coronary Procefs which stands up, and guards the Sigmoid Cavity before.

(4.) The Hollow, where the side of the smaller button-like head of the Radius rolls, called the Leffer Sigmoid Cavity.

(5.) The Prominent Roughnefs, into which the tendon of the Brachialis Internus is implanted; and it leads to the sharp ridge.

(6.) The Sharp Ridge, from which the Inter-offeous Membrane goes off.

(7.) The Lower Head of the Ulna, which is small, and button-like; for it is received into a hollow on the side of the Radius, and it is upon this point, viz. the little head of the Ulna, that the radius turns in the continual motions of the hand.

(8.) Is the Styloid Procefs of the Ulna, which is pointed, as the name implies; from it ligaments go off to strengthen the joint of the wrist.

FIGURE III.

EXPLAINS the relative pofition of the Radius and Ulna. The Ulna is marked with figures according with the above defcription; the Radius is alfo marked with its points of demonftration.

1. (*a. a. a.*)

1. (*a. a. a.*) Repeated on the three fides of the Radius, explain the general triangular form of the bone, marking particularly its three edges.

2. (*b*) Marks the upper head of the Radius, flat, round and button-like, with the fide rolling upon the Leffer Sygmoid Hollow of the Ulna.

3. (*c*) The neck of the Radius or ftraiter part, which immediately fupports the head.

4. (*d*) The Bump or Tubercle of the Radius, into which the tendon of the Biceps Mufcle is implanted.

5. (*e*) The Lower Head of the Radius; the Bone is thus gradually enlarging towards its lower end.

6. (*f*) The Scaphoid, or boat-like Cavity on the lower end of the Radius for receiving the two largeft bones of the Carpus ;—forming the wrift joint.

7. (*g*) The Styloid Procefs of the Radius, which bounds the wrift joint towards the fide of the thumb: and here it is seen how the little head of the Ulna (7) is received into the hollow focket on the fide of the Radius.——The two fharp edges of the Radius and Ulna are oppofed to each other, fhowing how the Inter-offeous Membrane ftretches from the one bone to the other, filling up all the fpace marked (*b*.) And it is here seen that the Radius is fomewhat arched towards the Ulna, fo as to roll round it without touching it, or hurting or difordering the numerous mufcles, &c. which lie upon the Inter-offeous Membrane.

FIGURE IV.

EXPLAINS the Bones of the CARPUS or WRIST, as they are feen from the outfide, or back of the hand.

The Bones of the Carpus are 8 in number, they are divided pretty regularly into two rows ;—and we rather choofe to count and demonftrate them according to their rank, than as individual and feparate bones : for as feparate bones there is nothing very particular in any one ; but by their combination and form, and as they relate to the

I   K   wrift wrist joint, or to the fingers, it surely must be important, I should rather say, neceſſary, for the ſurgeon to remember them.

- - -

FIRST ROW.

FORMING THE WRIST JOINT.

(1.) The Scaphoid Bone, where the figure (1.) marks the regular round ſurface, which forms a chief part of the ball and ſocket-joint of the wriſt. And (a) marks the great hook-like projection of this bone, whence that ſtrong ligament which braces down the tendons of the Carpus ariſes.

(2.) The Lunated Bone, where the figure is ſo placed as to mark the large ball-like ſurface of this bone which joins with the Os Scaphoides to form the ball of the wriſt. —— And the lunated part of the bone is concealed, when thus joined with the others.

(3.) The Cunieform Bone, of which only the broad or ſquare ſurface is ſeen on the back of the wriſt, while the narrower part of the wedge is in the palm.

(4.) The Piſiform Bone, ſo named from its roundneſs, this bone is a little removed from the direction of the row to which it belongs.

- - -

SECOND ROW.

RECEIVING THE METACARPAL BONES.

(5.) The Os Trapezium ; or firſt bone of the upper row named Trapezium, from its ſquare and angular form. It has the ball of the thumb planted upon, it and the figure points directly to that ſocket which receives the thumb,

(6.)

(6.) The Trapezoides, fo named from its refemblance to the laft.

(7.) Os Magnum, for it is the greateft; and it has a curious head which is in this view concealed under the Os Lunare; for the head of the Os Magnum is received into the femicircular hollow of the Os Lunare, forming a ball and focket joint with that bone.

(8.) The Os Unciforme, or hook-like bone; the hook of which is towards the palm, and therefore not feen in this view.

N. B. In this drawing of the Carpus, Fig. IV. this group of bones is made to reft chiefly upon two of the corner bones, viz. the hook of the Os Scaphoides, and the Os Pififorme.

FIGURE V.

IS alfo drawn chiefly with the intention of explaining the carpus; and here the fame numbers may ferve, for the pofition of the Carpus is very little changed.

(1.) is the Scaphoid Bone; (2.) The Lunar Bone, forming with the Scaphoid the ball for the wrift joint. (3.) The Os Cuneiforme. (4.) The Os Pififorme is out of fight. (5.) The Trapezium which fupports the thumb; (6.) (7.) (8.) The Trapezoides, Magnum, and Unciforme, fupporting all the others fingers; and here the Os Magnum (7.) is feen a little fuller; fo that the round head of it can almoft be feen jointed with the Os Lunare. The 1ft, 2d, and 3d Phallanges or rows of bones belonging to the feveral joints of the fingers, need not be explained; and the round heads for the joints of thefe finger bones explain themfelves.

FIGURE VI.

PRESENTS the Carpus in a new direction; fhowing thofe bones which are lefs perfectly feen in the other drawings;—and it is neceffary to obferve, that the group of the

I   K 2   Carpal

Carpal bones is now turned, fo as to fhow that face of them which receives the Metacarpal Bones;—and the group now refts chiefly upon the points of the two upper Corner Bones, *viz.* the Trapezoid and Unciform Bones; as in the other view it refted upon the lower Corner Bones, *viz.* the Scaphoid and Pifiform Bones. So that here there is only the upper row fairly demonftrated, *viz.*—(5.) The Os Trapezium;—(6.) the Os Trapezoides;—(7.) the Os Magnum;—(8.) the Os Un-ciforme. (*b*) Marks a fmall pointed projection of the Os Trapezium, whence the Carpal Ligament arifes.—(*c*) Marks the great Unciform or hook-like procefs of the Unciform Bone, which is another point whence the fame crofs ligament of the Carpus rifes.—(*d*) Marks the arch which the Carpal Bones make, and the Tendons of the wrift lie in this arch, and are bound down by the crofs ligament crofling from the one corner point, to the other.

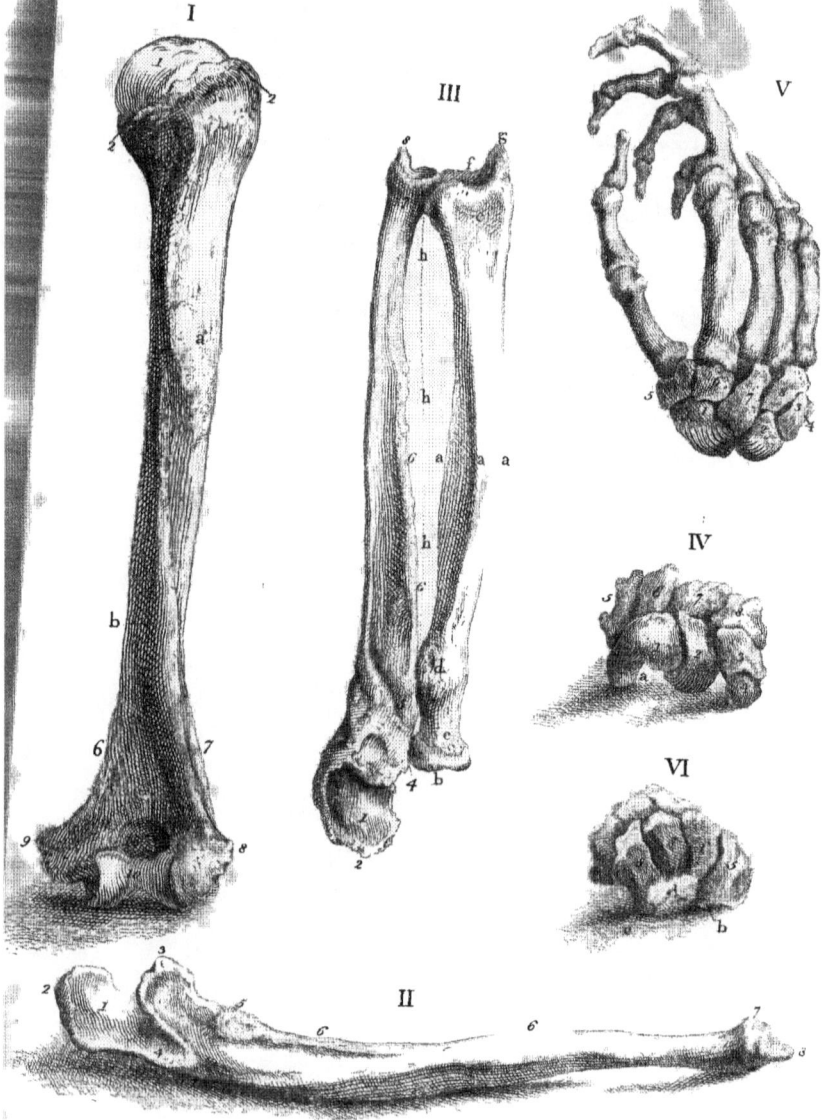

BONES

I

III

V

IV

VI

II

THE

SECOND BOOK.

OF THE

MUSCLES.

BOOK SECOND.

OF THE

MUSCLES.

— ·—

PLATE I.

MUSCLES OF THE FACE.

This Plate explains the Text Book, from page 191, *to page* 213.

THIS Plate explains the chief Muscles of the Face; and there are seen here several Muscles also of the Neck, Throat, Shoulder, and Breast.— It was drawn from a subject that had been hanged, and the neck being broken, the head lies flatter upon one shoulder, than it should do even in the dead body; for the Atlas and Dentatus, the two first Vertebræ of the Neck, were fairly broken loose from each other.—The Muscles are more distinctly seen on the left side; on the right side they are thrown into shadow, and are but faintly indicated.—The muscles of the outline are truer in point of Anatomy; while, in the full engraving, the

general

general appearance, the thinnefs and delicacy, and the undefined connections of the mufcles, are well expreffed ; and it is to be particularly
noticed, that the Levator Anguli Oris (7.) is not fo true in the engraving, while it is, I believe, very true and correct in the outline.

(1.) Is the Occipito Frontalis, which covers the Occiput and forehead, with its two
flefhy bellies, and the crown or top of the head with its thin flat tendon. The Occipital Belly is not feen here. The thin Tendon fometimes miftaken for the Pericra-
nium, is marked (*a*) ; the Frontal Belly is marked (*b*) ; or rather there are two
Frontal Bellies marked (*b b*). Each Frontal Belly fends a fmall flip of fibres, or a
peak, down upon the back of the Nofe marked (*c*) *. The Frontalis is connected
chiefly with the fkin, but little with the bone ; is chiefly for furling up and wrink-
ling the fkin of the forehead.

(2.) Is the Corrugator Supercilii, more connected with the Orbicularis Oculi,
than with the Occipito Frontalis, and lying under the Occipito Frontalis.

(3.) Is the Orbicularis Oculi ; arifing by a fmall white Tendon (*d*), from the Nafal
Procefs of the Jaw Bone. Its fibres go in regular circles round the eye, and they
are continued circles which return to the white Tendon in the corner of the eye,
whence they firft arife ; the whole mufcle is thin, flat, broad, very diftinct, fhuts
the eye-lids, compreffes the eye, fqueezes out the tears †.

The

* This Nafal Peak of the Occipito Frontalis is not the flip which is fixed into the Os Frontis ; that
lies deeper, while this Nafal Peak is fuperficial, runs down the back of the Nofe, expanding upon it,
and forming with the mufcles below a fort of fafcia, or Tendinous expanfion, which covers the Nofe
This Nafal flip is implanted rather into the fkin of the Nofe, and wrinkles it ; while the General
Mufcle corrugates the fkin of the forehead.

† The whole of what we call the Orbicularis Oculi, is named by Walther, Corrugator Oculi ;
and he feems to divide it into an upper and lower portion, by the names of Mufculus Semicircularis
Palpebræ Superioris, and Mufculus Semicircularis Palpebræ Inferioris.

The CORRUGATOR SUPERCILII (2.) arises from the Os Frontis betwixt the Eye-brows, and lies under that Peak of the FRONTALIS which expands upon the back of the Nose.— This Corrugator may almost be considered as merely a flip of the Orbicularis Oculi (3.); for in fact the fibres of the Corrugator go round the orbit with the upper fibres of the Orbicularis Oculi, and mix with them, so as to form the upper edge of the Orbicularis; and thence the names of Corrugator and Orbicularis are sometimes interchanged *.

(5.) † Is the LEVATOR LABII SUPERIORIS, and ALÆ NASI; This muscle arises by a small double Tendon, from the Nasal Process of the Upper Jaw Bone, and has one little flip (e) going into the Ala Nasi for dilating it; and another (f) going into the upper lip, for drawing it upwards ‡.

(6.) LEVATOR LABII SUPERIORIS PROPRIUS, arises from the Jaw Bone at the very edge of the Orbit, and above the Infra Orbitary Hole §. It has two flips of fibres, one (g) coming from the bone, from under the Orbicularis Muscle, and another flip, (h) which is continued from the lower fibres of the Orbicularis Muscle itself. So this is a Biceps Muscle; it lies superficially; it draws the middle of the lip upwards; it is often named as a Biceps or two headed Muscle ‖.

L

7. LEVATOR

* Walther, in his description of his own and Sanctorin's Plates, draws into the explanation of this Corrugator Muscle, all the upper part of the Orbicularis Oculi; as if it were but a part of the Corrugator.

† It will be observed here, that the suite of the numbers 1, 2, 3, &c. is not regularly followed, because it was impossible to explain absolutely every muscle in any sett of drawings, however full.

‡ "Maxime hunc in usum habent illi, qui detractores contemptoresque sunt aliorum, et forte hæc "verba in uno vel altero eundum motum excitabunt."

§ This is the MUSCULUS PYRAMIDALIS of Walther.

‖ Eustachius draws the muscle with these two heads. Albinus describes the little head (h), as a distinct part of the muscle, both in his explanation of Eustachius, and in his own plates. Cant observes

(7.) Levator Anguli Oris ; arifes above the dog tooth, and is thence named Caninus.—
This mufcle arifes under the Infra Orbitary Hole, as the laft arofe from above it ; this
of courfe lies under the laft, and fo is lefs perfectly feen here. Its direction is different
from that of the Levator Labii ; as it runs more perpendicularly, or runs rather
outwards than inwards. It is fhort ; two headed like the laft ; rifes properly from
the Socket Procefs of the firft Grinder. It lifts the Angle of the mouth, whence
its name ; and it operates on both lips, whence it is named, Levator Communis.

(8.) Zygomaticus Major ; arifes from the Zygomatic Procefs of the Cheek Bone ;
goes inwards to the corner of the mouth ; is long, flender, oblique in its direction.
It paffes over that hollow in the Cheek Bone, which is filled up with fat, and fo
when the mufcle is diffected, it falls into this loofe flaccid and bending form *.

(9.) The Zygomaticus Minor, like it, but not always found.

(10.) The Buccinator, is feen here to lie deeper ; it forms the flat part of the cheek ;
it arifes from the Coronoid Procefs of the Lower Jaw, and from the roots of the
back Grinders. It goes forward with direct fibres, (as feen here) towards the
corner of the mouth.

(11.) The Triangularis, is neat, fmall, triangular ; its bafe arifes from the Jaw, its
point ends in the corner of the mouth.—It draws the corner of the mouth down,
and is named Depreffor Anguli Oris, or the Depreffor Communis Labiorum.

(12.) Is the Depressor Labii Inferioris Proprius. This mufcle arifes from the line
of the Jaw, touches and croffes its fellow under the middle of the lower lip. They
pull the lip downwards.

(13.) The Orbicularis Oris, is thick, broad, and flefhy ; forms the flefhy part of the
                                                                        lip ;

ferves this feparate part proceeding from the fibres of the Orbicularis, fo particularly as to reckon it
almoft a diftinct mufcle, a depreffor of the lower Eye-lid ; faying, " Ex confpectu illum habere decet,
" pro depreffore Mufculo Palpebræ Inferioris." Cantü Impetus.

* This Zygomaticus Major, is fometimes fplit into two infertions at the angle of the mouth.

lip ; is in the red part of the lip, but is much broader than the red part. Its fibres are grofs and ftrong, they go in a circular direction fairly round both lips, they are not interrupted at the angles of the mouth ; they fend up a fmall flip, which paffing in the furrow of the lip, and mounting upon the Septum of the Nofe, is named Nafalis, and is marked (*i*).

(15.) The CONSTRICTOR NASI, is here diftinctly marked running over the point of the Nofe *.

(30.) Is the TEMPORAL MUSCLE ; which is feen here, lying under its fafcia. The fafcia, or Tendinous expanfion of the Temple being here entire, and nothing cut away but the Membraneous Mufcles of the ear, the ANTERIOR and the SUPERIOR AURIS.

(31.) Is the MASSETER, which is a fhort, thick, and flefhy mufcle ; and to lay it entirely open, the Parotid Gland which is marked (*k*), is diffected up from the cheek, fo that the head of the Maffeter is feen arifing from the Cheek Bone ; and its lower end is feen implanted into the Jaw †.

(*m*) Marks the FASCIAL ARTERY, or LABIAL ARTERY, as it is called, the Artery of the face, croffing over the angle of the Jaw.

Thus we fee in the dead body, thofe mufcles which give form and character to the human countenance, lying all dead and flaccid. The mouth open, the lips loofe and fhrivelled ; the angles of the mouth dropping down, the cheek funk ; and the eye alfo clofed, and funk down within its orbit.—All the countenance is deformed, and the traits of individual character or beauty, quite gone :—but ftill enough remains to explain to us what thofe mufcles are, upon which chiefly the interefting variety of expreffion and form depends. The Occipito Frontalis wrinkles the

L 2   forehead.

* This is the Tranfverfus Nafi of Walther. The action of this mufcle is very diftinctly feen, in the agony of an Afthmatic fit ; it is feen alfo in violent diftortion, produced by rage, or defpair. Cant compares it to that mufcle in the dog, by which he curls the Nofe, and fhows the teeth in fnarling.

† This is fometimes called, the MUSCULUS MANSOR.

forehead: the Corrugator Supercilii knits the brows: the Levatores Labiorum lift up the lip, fpread wide the noftrils, and open the mouth; the Depreffores Labiorum depress the lip; the Triangular Mufcles draw down the corners of the mouth; the Zygomatic Mufcle diftorts the cheek, and the Orbicularis Oris antagonifes all thefe, and clofes the mouth.—Thefe mufcles, while they are performing more important offices, alfo exprefs the paffions, and mark the countenance with traits never to be effaced, the true ftudy of thofe who would be Phyfiognomifts; who talk but idly, when they fpeak of expreffion in thofe immoveable features, which are formed rather by the Contour of a bone. " The fagacious forehead or œconomical " nofe," are the rhapfodies of an Enthufiaft, not the ferious obfervations of a fedate man, ftudious of that fubject, which is interefting above all others.

The fhapes of the bones determine the general form of the face. One great mufcle, the Mafieter, gives the rounding of the cheek; the reft are all delicate and moveable mufcles; and the great characters of the face, center round the mouth and noftrils where thefe mufcles converge. The lean and delicate face, gains in expreffion where the cheek is hollow, the angle of the mouth moveable, the lines ftrong; but in thofe who are bloated, the cheek is fuller, the lines obliterated, the delicate turnings of thought and feeling are loft; all but the more violent ftrains of paffion are burried in the mafs. The great lines of character, are the line of the Zygomatic Mufcle, coming from above, and of the Triangular Mufcle coming from the chin; and the moving point towards which they all act, is the corner of the mouth. In chearful emotions the features rife all towards the eye, which becomes full and turgid. In the depreffing paffions the features fink, the eye is languid, and the whole countenance gets a thoughtful ferious caft. But ftill it is the corner of the mouth, that is the central point of all thefe changes.

The corners of the mouth are continually fupported by the action of the Levator, and of the Zygomatic Mufcles; they are raifed high in fmiling, fo as to form a dimple there. They are raifed higher in laughter, fo as to fwell the cheek, wrinkle the

a   eye

eye-lids, and comprefs the eye, till tears begin to flow. And the corner of the mouth, which is thus raifed in laughter, is diftorted in pride, malice, hatred; is dilated and drawn backwards in rage; drops lower in grief; and in palfy falls quite down.

Thefe movements round the angle of the mouth, are the chief indications in the face itfelf, while all other indications of paffion, proceed rather from the general fyftem. A healthy body, and chearful mind, have the face full, the eye humid, the limbs braced, the whole body free, and light moving. In languid health, or under affliction and care, the face is pale, the eye cold, the whole body languid and relaxed ; and fo it is in paffion, for the medical arrangement of the paffions is nearly correct. There are two great claffes of paffions, the exciting and the depreffing paffions ; in the exciting paffions, as joy or anger, the heart beats high ; the face is turgid ; the eye prominent and fparkling ; the mufcles are tenfe ; the limbs braced ; the whole body is in a moveable, active, and highly excited ftate. But when the heart beats languid in grief, or palpitates with fear, the face becomes pale, the features fink, the limbs tremble, the whole frame is unbraced, cold, and unapt for motion ; and from thefe general conditions of the fyftem refult all thofe other marks of paffion, which accompany the changes of the face ; for in grief, fear, defpair, the blood ebbs, and the face is pale, and the features fink ; while in anger the face is red, the eye brows corrugated, and the eye turgid and ftrained ; but in rage, the whole mufcular frame is ftrained toward the moft violent action, the breath is retained, while the pulfe beats high ; and fo the face becomes turgid, the eye is fiery and red, there is a grinding of the teeth, the angles of the mouth are ftrained backwards, the noftrils are raifed and dilated, the Buccinator, Zygomatic, Maffeter, and Temporal Mufcles are in violent action, which gives an Angular and Linear hardnefs to all the features ; and faliva and foam proceed from the univerfal preffure upon all the glands.

MUSCLES

MUSCLES OF THE EYE.

FIGURES XII. AND XIII. of Plate II. Explain the Mufcles of the Eye.

The origin of the Mufcles at the bottom of the Orbit, being once underftood, all their mechanifm will be very plain and eafy, for this fingle point has been the chief diffi- culty from the firft. Galen counted the Levator Palpebræ, as one of the proper mufcles of the eye; Vefalius underftood better than Galen the origin of the Recti Mufculus from the bottom of the Orbit, but like Galen he has drawn the eye from Brutes, and has defcribed its mufcles, and drawn them in fo confufed a way, that it is not eafy to comprehend that mufcle of his, " which adheres in all its " courfe to the Optic Nerve. (Septimus Oculi Mufculus, nulla ex parte a viforio " nervo liberatus.") But even after this difcovery of the true origin of thefe mufcles, one author of very high reputation, Mr Lieutaud, denied the origin of thefe mufcles around the root of the Optic Nerve; believing that the fixed point, or center of all thefe mufcles, was a point a little to the outer fide of that hole, by which the Optic Nerve enters the focket.

But now this point, of their general origin from the bottom of the focket, is univerfally acknowledged; and the chief difpute is, whether thefe five mufcles, in arifing round the root of the Optic Nerve, begin from the periofteum of the focket; or from the bone itfelf, or from the outer coat (the Dura Mater) of the Optic Nerve; or whether they do not arife by a particular ring, which furrounds the root of the Optic Nerve; for Valfava believed that thefe mufcles began by a fort of ring, which as it furrounded the root of the Optic Nerve, he chofe to call Circulus Moderato- rius Nervi Optici. But in this difpute, as ufually happens, both parties are right, and both are in fome degree wrong; for two of the five mufcles arife more properly from the outer coat of the Optic Nerve, while the three others arife plainly from
the

the Dura Mater where it forms the periofteum of the Orbit; the Dura Mater gradually affuming the nature of a common tendon, from which thofe three mufcles
arife.

The place where this tendon begins, is the inner end of that Foramen Lacerum which
belongs to the Sphœnoid Bone, and which admits the fmaller nerves to enter for
the mufcles of the eye; for when the Dura Mater has come out by this hole from
the Cranium into the Orbit, it affumes, juft where it covers that hole, a hard and
tendinous nature, becomes white, affumes the appearance of a tendon, and is in
fact, the common Tendon by which three of the mufcles arife; and as this hole
is below the Optic Nerve, and toward the outer fide of it, the mufcles which arife
by this common tendon are chiefly thofe which pull the eye outwards or downwards; and fo this common tendon gives origin to the Abductor, Deprimens and
Adductor.

But thofe mufcles again which cover the upper part of the Optic Nerve, arife clofe
round the margin of the Optic hole; they touch the nerve and adhere to it; by adhering to the nerve, they may be faid to arife from the nerve or from that Angle
of the Dura Mater where it comes through the Optic hole, to go over the Optic
Nerve. So the Levator and the Obliquus Superior arife from the Dura Mater,
where it forms the fheath of the Optic Nerve; while the Deprimens, Abductor, and
Adductor, arife by one common tendon from the Dura Mater where it covers the
Foramen Lacerum, forming the periofteum of the orbit.

This is all feen at (a), Figures XII. and XIII. where (a) fhows the fringed edge of the
Dura Mater furrounding the root of the Optic Nerve; (b) the origins of the Levator
and Obliquus Superior, in the angle where the Dura Mater turns backwards. And
(c) fhows the origin of the Abductor and Deprimens coming from the Periofteum
of the Foramen Lacerum, a little to one fide of the great Nerve.

The only other difficult point, and which is more important ftill, fince it explains the
relative fize, and fhape, and courfe of thefe mufcles, is the true place of this
central

central point from which the mufcles rife, or in other words, the true place of
the Optic hole by which the Optic Nerve enters, and from the margins of which
all thefe mufcles rife. This will be eafily explained by the marginal plate, which
fhows the holes within the focket ; the pofition of the eye with regard to thofe
holes, and fo explains the relative length of each of the mufcles.

1ft, The eye is placed in the focket, as I have reprefented by the circle (a), not directly in the middle, but a little to one fide. The eye does not look out from the
Orbit in the direction of the Axis of the Orbit ; for the axes of the two orbits
meet almoft in the bottom of the focket, croffing in the Cella Turcica, * but
both the eyes look directly forwards. The plane of the fore part of the Orbit
being oblique, and falling off towards the temple, while the eye looks directly
forwards ; the axis of the Orbit, and of the eye can not coincide †. This is the
reafon of the Pupil, being nearer to one angle and not in the center of the focket,
for which we have the beft authority, that of meafuring the eye when we pleafe.
But the authorities of books on this point are thefe ; Heifter makes the Pupils
diftant three inches from each other. Camper makes the Pupils diftant two inches and a half. But the eye being compared not with the other eye, but with
its own focket, it is found that the center of the Pupil is eight lines from the outer
angle of the eye, and feven lines from its inner angle ‡. Thefe are my rules for
placing the eye in its focket, in this plan. And the eye being thus regularly
placed, we find by this drawing, (not geometrically true, but ftill fufficient for
proving and illuftrating fo plain a matter as this is,) that the Foramen Opticum
and the larger end of the Foramen Lacerum are much above the center of the
orbit, and towards the inner fide ; whence it is plain that the Optic Nerve in going
towards the ball of the eye, moves a little outwards and defcends. And it is alfo

very

* Camper.
† Winflow, Academie des Sciences.
‡ Petit Acadamie des Sciences.

very manifeſt, that ſince the muſcles, to get at their inſertions muſt go round the globe of the eye ; thoſe which go round by the outer ſide of the eye, or paſs under it, muſt be longer, while their antagoniſts which keep to the inner ſide of the eye or go over the globe, muſt be ſhorter. And ſo the Adductor Muſcle which is on the ſide next the noſe, is the only ſtraight muſcle ; it is the ſhorteſt, while the Abductor is the longeſt. The Abductor and the Deprimens Oculi, are the longer muſcles of the eye : The Adductor and the Levator Oculi, are the ſhorter muſcles.

In this plan, the center of the ſocket (*a*) is marked by the croſſing of its two diameters. The center of the Pupil is marked at (*b*) nearer the inner angle of the eye, the Foramen Opticum is marked (*c*), and the inner end of the Foramen Lacerum is marked (*d*).

M   In

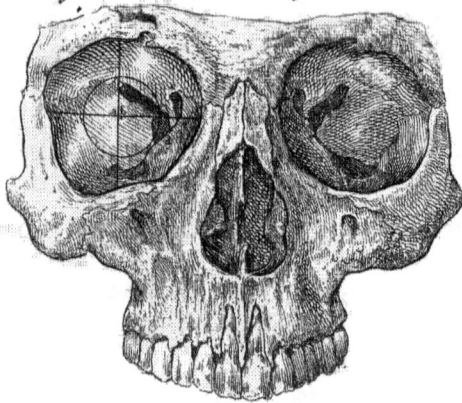

Plan for the Muscles of the Eye

In Figure XII. these points are seen ; (a) the ring which the Dura Mater forms, where
it comes from the brain into the Orbit, accompanying the Optic Nerve ; (b) the origin of the Obliquus Superior and Levator, from this part of the Dura Mater furrounding the Optic Hole. (c) The origins of the Abductor and Deprimens, but the
letter (c) points more particularly to the origin of the Abductor, which is here seen
to be a Biceps, or two headed muscle, having two Tendons, and the smaller nerves
which belong to the muscles of the eye are seen at (d), passing betwixt these two tendinous origins of the Abductor. For it is to be remembered, that this Abductor
along with two of the Recti, rises from that part of the Dura Mater, which covers
the Foramen Lacerum ; and that the small nerves enter the socket by the Foramen Lacerum.

From this root round the Optic Nerve, the muscles are seen going forwards.

1. The Obliquus Superior or Trochlearis (29) uppermost, the longest muscle of the
   eye with its slender Tendon passing through the Cartilaginous Pulley (e), which is
   left still in its place attached to the Superciliary Ridge of the Frontal Bone (f).

2. The Obliquus Inferior, (30) is seen, the shortest muscle of the eye, arising from
   the lower part of the Orbit, and going backwards to antagonize the last.

3. The Rectus Superior (25) next to the Rectus Internus which it hides, is the
   shortest muscle.

4. The Rectus Externus (28) or Abducens Oculi, is the longest of all the straight
   muscles of the eye.

5. The Rectus Inferior or Deprimens Oculi (26) is shorter than the Abducens, (28)
   but longer than the Rectus Superior (25), because the Optic Nerve enters a little
   above the center of the Orbit. The Tendons of these Recti Muscles are seen expanding flat and broad upon the forepart of the eye ; where by shining through that thin
   and Transparent skin, which covers the forepart of the eye, they form what is called
   the Albuginia, or white coat of the eye.

There

There remains but one mufcle belonging to the eye, and that is, the LEVATOR PALPE-
BRÆ SUPERIORIS (4); which is explained in FIGURE XIII. where it is feen rifing
from the upper part of the Optic Hole at (a), along with the other mufcles; it
lies over all the other mufcles, and expands into a thin and membraneous flefh (b),
which runs imperceptibly into the fubftance of the upper eye-lid; and feems to
end in (c) the Tarfus, or Cartilaginous hoop of the eye-lid.

The XIV FIGURE of this plate, explains the mufcles of the outward ear, as they are
exprefled by COWPER. Where (17) marks the SUPERIOR AURIS or Atollens; and
(19) the POSTERIOR AURIS or Retrahens, as they are explained in the book of the
mufcles, p. 240. 204.

M 2   P L A T E

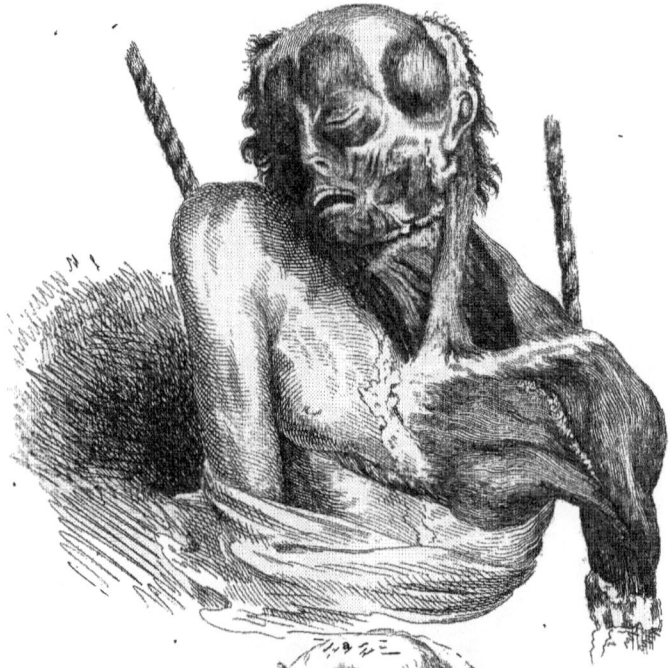

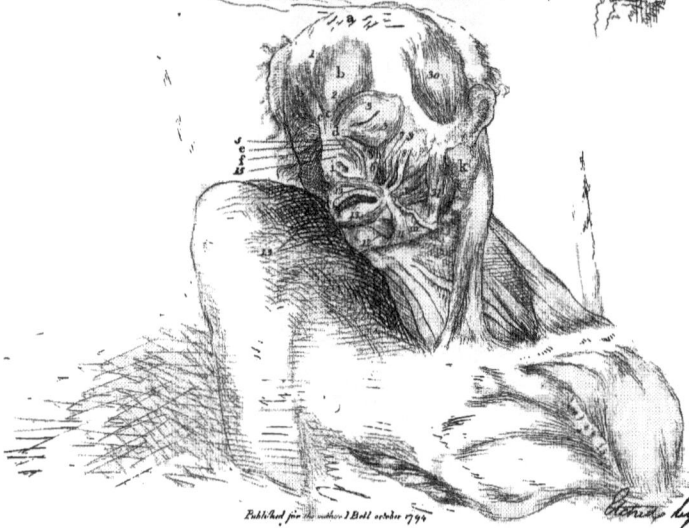

Publish'd for the author J Bell october 1794

P L A T E II.

This Plate explains the Text Book, from page 212, to page 231.

THIS plate belongs chiefly to the Throat; explains the Cartilaginous and bony parts, of which the upper part of the throat and efpecially the flute part or Larynx is formed; fhows the Os Hyoides; the Thyroid, Cricoid, and Arytenoid Cartilages; the Epiglottis; and the Membranes and Mufcles by which thefe Cartilages are connected, fo as to form a rigid tube confifting of parts moveable upon one another, and yet fo firm upon the whole, as to be a protection to all the more delicate parts of the throat, and to be the center of all the motions of the Jaws, and Tongue, and Windpipe, and Gullet; or of the Larynx and Pharynx, as they are called.

THIS Plate explains firft all the individual parts one by one; and then joins them, fhowing how the whole is compofed; without which regular form of demonftration, nothing could be clearly underftood of parts fo very intricate and difficult, and having fo long a catalogue of hard names connected with them.

2   FIRST

———————

FIRST ROW.

The firft row gives the parts fingle and entirely diffected; and there is reprefented,

(1.) The Os Hyoides, which refembles in its general form the lower Jaw Bone of a
child, or what is called the Thought Bone of a fowl; (a) is its bafis, (b) its horn,
(c) the Cartilaginous joinings of the horns and body, and two little Tubercles
ftand perpendicularly up at the place of this joining, which are called the
Cornua Minora or leffer horns, or Appendices of the Os Hyoides. Thefe Cornua Minora are here reprefented in outline. The Os Hyoides is named alfo the
bone of the Tongue, and its connections are efpecially to be obferved, *viz.* that
it lies in the root of the tongue; forms in a manner the top piece of the Trachea,
is tied by a membrane to the Thyroid Cartilage, has the Epiglottis (5.) or valve
of the windpipe planted upon it. And that thefe connections may be underftood,
this bone is marked with this figure (1.) in all the other drawings.

(2.) Is the Thyroid or Shield-like Cartilage; which is indeed the fhield of the
Throat, for it is broad, flat, and very deep, and a full inch in length; it is thick,
and often offified. And accordingly it is this broad Cartilage that defends the more
delicate parts; its upper horns (dd), are tied to the Os Hyoides by a long ligament; its lower ones (ee) clofely embrace the Cricoid Cartilage. In this drawing,
the Cartilage is fet fo as to reft upon its two lower Cornua, and to fupport and bal-
lance it a common pin marked (*), was thruft into it.

(3.) Is the Cricoid Cartilage; which is not, like the Thyroid, a femicircle merely,
i. e. wanting at the back part, but is an entire ring which forms, as it were, the
uppermoft and firmeft ring of the Trachea, but which ftill belongs properly to
the Larynx. It is fhallow before, and very deep in the back part of its circle,
plainly for the purpofe of raifing the Arytenoid Cartilages, (thofe fmall Cartilages
which

which form the Rima Glottidis or opening of the windpipe) ; and by this deepnefs at its back part, the Cricoid Cartilage raifes the opening of the Glottis fo high, (as is feen figures vii. and viii.) that it is behind the very center of the Thyroid Cartilage where it is well defended and fafe. The Articulating Surfaces upon which the Arytenoid Cartilages fit down, are marked (*f*).

(4.) The ARYTENOID CARTILAGES, are the fmall and moveable ones, which are of a Triangular form; they are fet down upon the upper border of the Cricoid Cartilage, by their bafe (*g*) with a very moveable articulation ; and (*g*) points to the focket furface of the Arytenoid Cartilage by which the articulation is formed. For here the two uppermoft drawings of the Cartilage are fet oppofite to each other, almoft in their natural pofitions, and refting upon their bafis, while the loweft drawing of the three, is turned up fo as to fhow its joint. The two fharp points of the Arytenoid Cartilages ftand perpendicularly upwards, and give the fhape and opening of the Glottis. The tips of the two Arytenoid Cartilages are feen over the Thyroid Cartilage in figure vii . and the Cartilages are feen full in figure viii, fettled in their place, and forming the Rima Glottidis or chink of the windpipe, which is narrower or wider as they are moved by their mufcles.

(5.) Shows the Epiglottis, which may be compared to an Artichoke leaf. It flaps down like a fmall tongue or valve, and, by clapping neatly down upon the Rima Glottidis, makes the food and drink glide clear over the Glottis, and into the Gullet or Pharynx. The Epiglottis is reprefented in this drawing, fo as to explain its connection with the Os Hyoides, and of courfe with the root of the tongue.

SECOND ROW.

The connections are explained in the figures of the fecond row ; each part preferves its peculiar marks (1. 2. 3.) &c. and it is feen in figure vi. in what fucceffion thefe parts ftand.

(1.) The

FIGURE   VI.

(1.) The Os Hyoides, connected by its long horns with the upper horns of the Thyroid Cartilage. It is a ligament (*b*) of a full inch in length that connects them. And the common membrane of the Trachea is continued from the Os Hyoides, to the Thyroid Cartilage, so that the gap betwixt them is filled up by a strong, but thin membrane (*i*).

(2.) The Thyroid Cartilage is next, it stands forwards in the throat to defend the other parts; is distinctly felt without; is the most prominent part of the throat; and named Pomum Adami.

(3.) Is the Cricoid Cartilage, which in this profile of the throat, is seen to be very shallow before, as it is deep behind.

The Arytenoid Cartilages, (4.) are necessarily hidden in this view; and the Epiglottis (5.) is cut away, to make this drawing more simple and easy.

The Thyroid Gland is marked (6.) the chief part of it is seen on the nearer side of the Trachea, and a part also of the right lobe is seen coming round from the other side behind the Trachea, and almost surrounding it. (7.) Marks the Trachea, and the figure is here made to point to the uppermost ring, that the true place of the Thyroid Gland might be understood, for it lies not upon the Thyroid Cartilage (2.) nor upon the Cricoid Cartilage (3.) as might be supposed, but upon the second ring of the Trachea, leaving the first one free.

FIGURE   VII. AND VIII.

Are chiefly useful in explaining the places of the two Arytenoid Cartilages, and the way in which they form the opening of the Glottis.

FIGURE VII. The Os Hyoides is cut away. The Thyroid Cartilage (2.) is seen in

its

its place, defending and concealing the Arytenoid Cartilages; or at least the tips only of the Arytenoid Cartilages are seen (4.) peeping over the border of the Thyroid Cartilage. (3.) The fore-part of the ring-like or Cricoid Cartilage, is seen connected with the upper ring of the Trachea; but leaving an interstice (*k*) of a triangular form, at which point, (and not betwixt the rings of the Trachea), Mr Vique D. Azir proposes to perform the operation of Bronchotomy.

FIGURE VIII. Shows the back view of the same dissection. The Os Hyoides is shown in outline, and in its true position with its small ligament which connects it with the upper horns of the Thyroid Cartilage; and here it is explained how (1. 1.) the two horns of the Os Hyoides project far beyond the Larynx. They belong more properly to the Pharynx, " and hold the Pharynx extended, as we " hold a bag open with the finger and thumb."

(2. 2.) Show how deep the Thyroid Cartilage is; how fairly it inclofes the Cricoid Cartilage, and conceals and defends the Arytenoid Cartilages and the opening which they make; and here it is seen, that the edges of the Thyroid Cartilages belong also to the Pharynx, for the borders of the Thyroid Cartilage do, in fact, form part of the sides of the Pharynx; they assist the horns of the Os Hyoides, in keeping the bag of the Pharynx extended. And the Constrictor Pharingis, (44. 45. 46.) the great Circular Muscle which embraces the Pharynx, arises chiefly from the tips of the horns of the Os Hyoides, and from this projecting edge of the Thyroid Cartilage.

(3.) Is seen the great deepness of the Cricoid Cartilage behind, and it is seen by (4.), how the Glottis (which is just the opening betwixt the two Arytenoid Cartilages), is raised by this deepness of the Cricoid Cartilage, in its back parts.

The third row of figures exhibits the more important of those delicate muscles by which the Cartilages are moved upon each other; but before these muscles are explained, it is necessary to observe the place and effect of the Epiglottis, which is well seen in figure x. and by the assistance of this figure joined with the de-

N   monstration

monstration of figure vi. the succeſſion of parts is very fairly explained.—1. The Os Hyoides.—2. The Thyroid Cartilage.—3. The Cricoid Cartilage follow each other in figure vi.—4. The Arytenoid Cartilages, figure vii. and viii.—5. The Epiglottis, figure ix.—6. The Thyroid Gland, figure vi.—7. The rings of the Trachea, betwixt which rings, and below the Thyroid Gland, the operation of Bronchotomy is to be performed.

This x. figure then compleats thoſe connections of the parts of the throat; and the effects of accidental wounds, or of the attempts of Suicides, or of our operation of Bronchotomy will be eaſily underſtood. Suicides in their attempts very commonly cut ſo high in the throat, immediately under the jaw, that they ſeldom wound the Carotid Artery; nor do they even hurt the more material parts of the throat; for they ſtrike ſo high, (commonly above the Thyroid Cartilage), that they do not touch the Trachea, nor injure the Glottis. They only cut off the Os Hyoides from the Larynx; they do not ſo properly cut the throat as the tongue; and when the food paſſes by the wound, it does not come from a cut of the Œſophagus acroſs the Trachea, but comes merely from the root of the tongue.

Theſe Lateral views explain alſo how idle it is to talk of performing Bronchotomy above the Thyroid Cartilage, ſince the Thyroid Cartilage is not in the Trachea, and ſince the obſtruction is below that point, being commonly in the Thyroid Gland, which is here marked (6).—Mr Vique D' Azir is not more correct in his Anatomy, where he adviſes Bronchotomy to be performed betwixt the Thyroid and Cricoid Cartilages, in the Triangular Membranous ſpace marked (k): for, that is exactly by the ſide of the Sacculus Laryngis, or Sac of the Larynx, a mucous ſecreting bag, which lies here on the inſide of the Trachea; and the Trocar would lie almoſt in the opening of the Glottis, or ſo near it, that the irritation could not be endured. The Larynx cannot bear the operation of Bronchotomy, becauſe it is moveable, furniſhed with many muſcles that are eaſily excited; and the leaſt irritation near the Glottis, throws them into violent contractions. But the Trachea itſelf, can eaſily bear to be

transfixed

transfixed with the Trocar, which neither excites contractions, nor gives pain : Befides the obftruction which requires Bronchotomy, is feldom in the tongue or mouth ; more commonly in the Larynx ; not unfrequently in the Thyroid Gland. So that almoft all the occafions that can be fuppofed, are fuch as keep us down to the very loweft point of the Trachea, *viz.* That neareft the cheft.

THIRD ROW.

This row is for demonftrating the chief mufcles of the Larynx, and Pharynx ; and of courfe, the motions of thefe feveral parts upon each other. And it explains, firft, the mufcles which lie immediately upon the Cartilages of the Larynx, and which move the parts of the throat upon each other ; and thefe lead to a knowledge of thofe longer mufcles, which come from the jaws, or chin, or fternum, or fhoulder ; and by which the whole throat is moved. Thefe are reprefented carefully in the middle figure of this third row, and alfo in the next plate.

FIGURE IX. Explains chiefly the Hyo-thyroidæi, and Crico-thyroidæi Mufcles ; for firft, The CRICO-THYROIDÆI (42), arife by a fmall pointed origin, (*l*) from tho fore part of the Cricoid Cartilage ; go upwards and obliquely outwards about an inch in length ; are implanted by a broad infertion (*m*), into the lower border of the Thyroid Cartilage, and where they end, the next mufcle begins. For the HYO-THYROIDÆUS (41), is a long, flat, and flefhy mufcle, about an inch and a half, or two inches in length ; lying flat upon the fmooth face of the Thyroid Cartilage ; rifing from the lower border of the Thyroid Cartilage below, and implanted broad and flefhy above, into the bafis of the Os Hyoides a little to one fide, and to a part of the horn. Sometimes this mufcle is divided into two flips, as it is drawn by Cowper, but more commonly it is fingle, as reprefented here, and the upper end of the Sterno-hyoideus (34), is feen here marked with its proper number.

N 2   The

The Sterno-*Thyroideus* is implanted into the Thyroid Cartilage, at the point where the Crico-thyroideus (42) ends, and the Hyo-thyroideus (41) begins; so that the Crico-thyroidæus is in part covered by the Sterno-thyroideus; and the Hyo-thyroideus again looks like a continuation of the same muscle.

In FIGURE X. are seen chiefly the small muscles by which the Cartilages of the Larynx are moved upon each other, modulating the voice. And the chief of these are, first, the CRICO-ARYTENOIDEUS POSTICUS, and secondly the ARYTENOIDEUS TRANSVERSUS.

The Crico-arytenoideus Posticus (45), " is a small Pyramidal Muscle, which rises " broader from the back part of the Cricoid Cartilage, where the ring is broad " and deep; and going directly upwards, is implanted with a narrow point into the " back of the Arytenoid Cartilage. This pair of muscles pulls the Arytenoid " Cartilages" backwards and outward, so that they at once lengthen and widen the slit; enlarging the opening of the Glottis. Under this lies the Crico-arytenoideus Lateralis, the smallest of these muscles, which arises from the rim of the Cricoid, and is inserted into the root of the Arytenoid Cartilage, and plainly separates the Arytenoid Cartilages, and widens the Glottis.

The ARYTENOIDEUS TRANSVERSUS, (43) is seen here. It is seen crossing betwixt the two Arytenoid Cartilages, going from the root of the one, to the root of the other; its natural office being to contract, or occasionally to close the Glottis.

The ARYTENOIDEUS OBLIQUUS, is a very delicate muscle which lies under this, in the same way that the Arytenoideus *Lateralis* lies under the Arytenoideus Posticus *.

The XI. FIGURE explains the Constrictores Pharyngis, and the Styloid Muscles; for (n) represents the Velum Pendulum Palati, cut off from the roof of the mouth, and

* The young student should carry the throat to his room, wash it in a hand bason, steep and dissect there.—A piece of Anatomy, which with these drawings he will easily manage, which is hardly uncleanly, and cannot but be very important. It is indeed neglected only from being thought impracticable.

and hung out by ftrings; (*o*) is the UVULA or Pap, in the centre of it; (*p*) is the Anterior Arch of the Palate; (*q*) is the Pofterior Arch; (*r*) is the Tonfil lurking betwixt the arches at the fide of the root of the tongue; (*s*) is the tongue; (1.) is the Os Hyoides; (2.) is the Thyroid Cartilage; (3.) the Cricoid Cartilage; (6) the Thyroid Gland; (*t*) the Trachea; (*u*) a piece of wood thruft up through the Œfophagus, and appearing again in the throat at the back part of the tongue; and the great conftrictor mufcle, is feen going in waves round this piece of wood; or in other words, courfing round the upper part of the Œfophagus, *i. e.* the Pharynx; and (*v*) is the laft point of this demonftration, and the moft important, for it is the Styloid Procefs, whence (39.) (53.) and (58.) the three Styloid Mufcles arife *.

The mufcles then which are to be feen in this drawing of the throat are, 1. The fet of the three Styloid Mufcles; 2. the Conftrictor Pharyngis; and 3. the Vaginalis Gulæ.

The Styloid Mufcles are, the STYLO-GLOSSUS (58.) arifing from the forepart of the Styloid Mufcle, and going forwards into the fubftance of the tongue, ftretching forwards into its point for drawing it back into the mouth.

The STYLO-HYOIDEUS (39), which begins rather from the backpart of the Styloid Procefs, and goes here into the fide of the Os Hyoides, being flender at its beginning, and broad towards its infertion, as all the Styloid Mufcles are.

The STYLO-PHARINGEUS (53.) lies behind or under the Stylo-hyoideus; for it lies clofe upon the Gullet or Pharynx, expands upon that part of the bag where it is held extended upon the horns of the Os Hyoides; fo that the Stylo-pharyngeus, when it expands upon the Pharynx, touches the horn of the Os Hyoides, which is marked (*x*), and as the middle conftrictor of the Pharynx arifes efpecially from

that

---

* The Stylo-gloffus I had defcribed in my book of the mufcles; but after claffing it in the general arrangement, I had forgotten it in the defcription of individual mufcles.

that point of the Os Hyoides, the lower fibres of the Stylo-pharyngeus run along-
side of the upper fibres of the middle conſtrictor, ſo that they almoſt mix.

Theſe three Styloid Muſcles perform the firſt movement in the act of ſwallowing,
for they all coincide in lifting up the throat, preſſing back the root of the tongue
againſt the palate, (to ſtraiten the Arches of the Fauces;) and confining the morſel.
By compreſſing the morſel, they puſh it down, and ſo begin that action, which is
compleated by that ſtrong Muſcle of the Pharynx, which is next ſeen.

For the CONSTRICTOR PHARYNGIS, (55.) is a very large and fleſhy muſcle, which covers
five inches (in length) of the Œſophagus, and puſhes down the morſel, which is
already preſſed by the contractions about the top of the Pharynx, and chiefly by
the action of the Styloid Muſcles. The Conſtrictor is fairly enough divided into
three muſcles, (54. 55. and 56.) of which the upper one, which cannot be ſeen here,
riſes about the back of the jaws, and from the baſis of the ſkull, and from the
root of the tongue.

The MIDDLE CONSTRICTOR, marked (55.) riſes from tips of the horns of the Os Hyoides
alone, and goes in a diverging form upwards, till it almoſt touches the ſkull, and
downwards pretty low upon the Gullet.

The LOWER CONSTRICTOR (56.) ariſes from the borders or wings of the Thyroid
Cartilage, and from the ring of the Cricoid Cartilage. This is the thickeſt and
fleſhieſt of all the Conſtrictors; it is very large, and goes obliquely upwards,
covering the lower part of the middle Conſtrictor, and a ſmall ſpace is left, a
kind of angle betwixt the two Conſtrictors, which is thin and membranous,
and there the tips of the horns belonging to the Thyroid Cartilage, are faintly
indicated, as ſhining through the thin membrane.

The ŒSOPHAGUS is ſtill farther covered with a ſheath of muſcular fibres, which run in
a perpendicular direction longitudinally along it, till they expand at laſt upon
the ſtomach itſelf. This ſheath of muſcular fibres is called the VAGINALIS GULÆ,
and is marked (57.)

P L A T E

Pl. II.

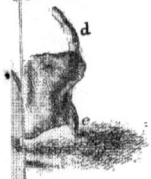
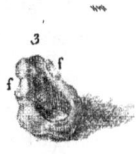
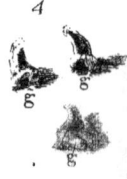
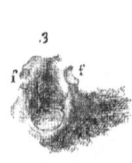
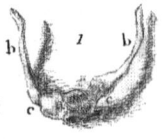

VIII VI VII

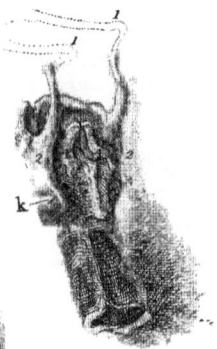
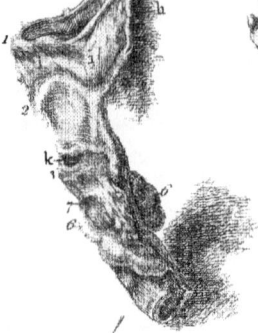
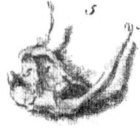
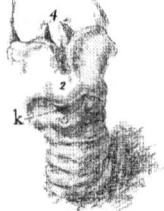

IX XI X

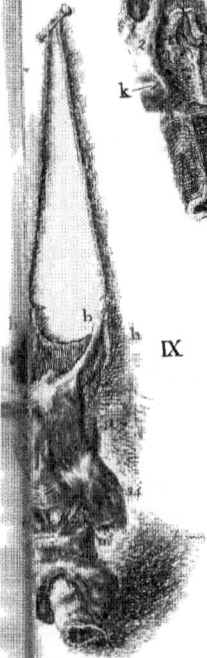
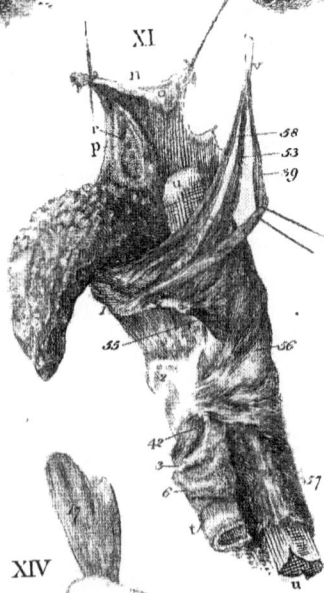
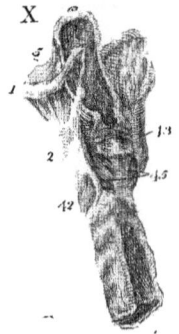

XIII XIV XII

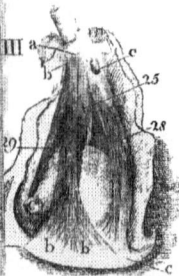
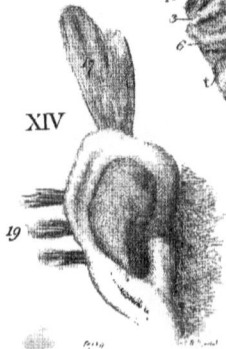
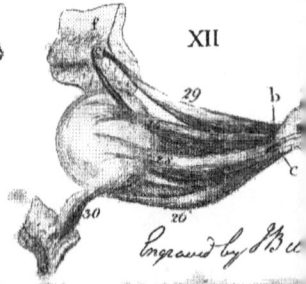

Engraved by J.B.

P L A T E   III.

This Plate explains the Text Book, from page 217. to page 220.

THIS Plate explains the connection of the muscles of the throat; it explains chiefly the greater muscles coming upwards from the breast and shoulder; or downwards from the Styloid Process, pulling the throat upwards towards the jaws, or downwards towards the Sternum; and these muscles, though they belong chiefly to the throat, do occasionly move the jaws.

IN FIGURE I. which represents the head of an old man, the skin of the neck is dissected off, and cut away, nearly in the line of the Jaw Bone; so as to show, (*a*) the Jaw Bone; (*b*) the Parotid Gland, lying behind the angle of the jaw; (*c*) the Submaxillary Gland, lying under the corner of the jaw; (*d*) the Great Carotid Artery, which carries blood to the head; (*e*) the Great Jugular Vein, by which that blood is returned; *g*) is the Thyroid Gland, which consists of two lobes, one lying upon the right side of the Trachea, the other upon the left side, the two lobes are joined by a narrow slip of the Glandular substance which lies upon the fore-part of the Trachea, and is called the ISTHMUS, *i. e.* neck betwixt the two lobes, joining together the two lobes of the Gland. The Gland is large, where the bulk of it can lie at either side of the Trachea; but its Isthmus marked (*g*) is very thin, and almost

membranous,

membranous, where it lies upon the fore-part of the Trachea. We find the Gland ſmaller in men, larger in women; of great variety in reſpect of ſize; very generally ſo large, as to be diſtinguiſhed by the fingers on the outſide of the throat; very often enlarged, and often deſcending deep behind the Trachea, ſo that the two oppoſite lobes almoſt meeting behind, ſurround that Tube, and explain to us how terrible and how incurable (by any operation at leaſt), that ſuffocation muſt be, which proceeds from a ſwelling of this Gland. This form of the Gland almoſt ſurrounding the Trachea, the two oppoſite lobes nearly meeting behind, is better explained in the Trachea, drawn at Figure vi. Plate ii.

The parts of the Trachea, with which the muſcles are more immediately connected; are,

(1.) The Os Hyoides, which lies in the root of the tongue.

(2.) The Thyroid Cartilage, where it projects to form the Pomum Adami.

(3.) The Cricoid Cartilage, which is above the Thyroid Gland. Therefore the Thyroid Gland is hardly entitled to the name of THYROID, ſince, in place of reſting upon the Thyroid Cartilage, it lies quite below both the Thyroid and Cricoid Cartilages, upon the firſt, or rather upon the ſecond ring of the Trachea.

THE MUSCLES ARE THESE,

(137.) is the STERNO MASTOIDEUS, the great muſcle of the neck; thrown back to expoſe thoſe ſmaller muſcles which belong properly to the throat; and there is ſeen,

(34.) The STERNO-HYOIDEUS, coming up from the Sternum, going upwards to the Os Hyoides, long, flat, ribband-like, and bending where it paſſes over the Thyroid Gland.

(35.) The STERNO-THYROIDEUS, coming alſo upwards from the Sternum; ſtretching towards the Thyroid Cartilage; lying under the laſt uamed muſcle; like it flat and ribband-like; covering alſo the Thyroid Gland, and bulging a little where it paſſes over the chief bulk of the Gland.

(36.) The OMO-HYOIDEUS, coming upwards from the ſhoulder. It is a digaſtric or
two-bellied

two-bellied mufcle. The belly (36.) is fixed into the Os Hyoides. The middle tendon (h) is feen under the Maftoid mufcle; and the lower flefhy belly lies too deep to
be feen, for it rifes from the Scapula near the Coracoid Procefs.

Thefe are the chief mufcles which pull the throat DOWNWARDS.

The mufcles which pull the throat UPWARDS are the MYLO-HYOIDEUS, the BIVENTER,
and the STYLO-HYOIDEUS mufcles.

(37.) The MYLO-HYOIDEUS arifes from the whole length of the Jaw Bone, from the
chin to the angle; and it arifes not from the lower border of the jaw; but rather from the inner furface of the jaw-bone, almoft as high as the fockets for the
teeth. It is thick and flefhy; but ftill it is flat and broad; and goes downwards in
a radiated or fan-like form, to be implanted into the bafis of the Os Hyoides.
Within this mufcle lies hidden the Genio-Hyoideus; without, lies the fore belly of
the Digaftric Mufcle; the Sub-maxillary Gland (c) is an external Gland, and lies
under the corner of the jaw without, (i. e.) over the Mylo-hyoideus; the Sub-
lingual Gland is an internal Gland which lies under the tongue beneath this mufcle.
The Mylo-hyoidei mufcles of oppofite fides are united to each other by a rapha or
tendinous feam or line, which is feen at (i), and which goes down from the center of
the chin to the center of the Os Hyoides.

(40.) The BIVENTER MAXILLÆ INFERIORIS belongs after all more properly to the throat
than to the jaw; it is called Biventer from its two bellies, which are indeed very diftinct and beautiful; one belly (k) arifes from the root of the Maftoid Procefs, and
fo is feen here coming out from under the Parotid Gland; the fore-belly (l) is feen
arifing from under the chin; the middle tendon has the number of the mufcle (40.)
put upon it at that point where it paffes the fide of the Os Hyoides, and there it is
attached to the Os Hyoides, not merely by running through a fort of Cartilaginous
loop on the fide of that bone, but alfo by running through a loop made by the flefh
of the Stylo-Hyoideus mufcle, which forks at its infertion.

(39.) Is the STYLO-HYOIDEUS coming from under the Parotid Gland, and implanted in-

to

to the fide of the Os Hyoides, and fo binding down the middle tendon of the digaftric mufcle.

In this drawing then, are feen the chief mufcles which affect the general pofition of the
throat, *viz.*

1. The Sterno-Hyoideus (34.), Sterno-Thyroideus (35.), and the Omo-Hyoideus,
   (36.) pulling the throat downwards.
2. The Mylo-Hyoideus (37.), the Stylo-Hyoideus (39.), and the Digaftricus (40.),
   pulling the throat upwards.

One fmall mufcle remains to be explained; it is the Crico-thyroideus (42.), which a-
rifes from (3.) the Cricoid Cartilage to be inferted into (2.) the Thyroid Cartilage.

FIGURE II.

Is the head of a woman, the neck long, the flender mufcles of the throat much diffected
and thrown out, very loofe and flaccid; and the Thyroid Gland was in this fubject
particularly large, hung very low down, and made a confiderable bending in the two
long mufcles which run over it. This drawing is a freer diffection of thefe
mufcles, where all the Anatomy of the throat is feen; for the Parotid Gland, the
Carotid Artery, the Jugular vein, the eighth pair of nerves, and the chief mufcles
both of the throat, and of the tongue, are here.

The Jaw Bone is here, as in the former figure, marked (*a*); the Parotid Gland (*b*);
the Carotid Artery (*d*); the Jugular vein (*e*); and the Thyroid Gland, which
appears only at two points, and almoft covered by the mufcles, is marked (*g*).
But the moft important parts in the Anatomy of the neck, are the Carotid Artery
(*d*); the Jugular vein (*e*); and the Par Vagum, or eighth pair of nerves (8.) This
eighth pair is a long nerve, which goes from the head down to the ftomach to end
there. It is marked (8.); it is feen here, lying upon the great Jugular vein, which

is

is turgid with blood, and bulging out in the form of a dilated inteftine : the eighth pair of nerves goes down along with the Carotid Artery and Jugular vein, they being all inclofed in one common fheath of Cellular Subftance, which is here diffected away, to fhow thefe parts clean.

The Os Hyoides is marked (1.); the Thyroid Cartilage is marked (2.); the Cricoid Cartilage is hidden by the mufcles.

In this drawing, the Sterno-maftoideus (137.) is very fully diffected, is made flaccid, and is laid to one fide, fo as to fhow the mufcles of the throat freely ; which for the fake of a clear demonftration, I fhall divide into three fets. 1. The mufcles from the Sternum, which pull the throat downwards. 2. The Digaftric and the Styloid Mufcles, which pull the throat upwards. 3. The mufcles which make the flefh of the tongue, the chief part of its bulk.

I. The mufcles coming upwards from the Sternum and fhoulder are,

(34.) The Sterno-hyoideus, which is feen in all its length, ftretching from the Sternum to the Os Hyoides, and bending over the Thyroid Gland.

(35.) The Sterno-thyroideus ; exactly like this, lying behind and under it, proceeding from the Sternum to end in the Thyroid Cartilage, and alfo bending over the Thyroid Gland.

(41.) Is the place where the Sterno-thyroideus ends ; and the Thyro-hyoideus begins ; this (41.) then, is like a continuation of the fame mufcle, while it is really a diftinct one, named Thyro-hyoideus (41.) becaufe it goes from the Thyroid Cartilage, to the Os Hyoides.

(36.) Is the Omo-hyoideus, of which the flefhy belly is marked, as in the other drawing (36.) while its middle tendon is marked (b).

2. The

II. The muscles which pull the throat upwards are,

(40.) The Digastricus, of which the first belly (40.) is seen coming out from under the Thyroid Gland, while the fore belly (*n*) being cut away from the chin, hangs down.

(39.) The Stylo-Hyoideus Muscle, which is seen turning over the tendon of the Digastricus, and tying it down in its place.

(53.) The Stylo-pharyngeus, which lies very deep behind the other Styloid Muscles, passes down under the arm or branch of the Os Hyoides, and expands upon the Pharynx.

N. B. In this drawing, the Styloid Muscles are dissected upwards very nearly to that point (under the Parotid Gland,) where they rise small and delicate, from around the roots of the Styloid Procefs.

III. The muscles which compose the chief bulk of the tongue, are these,

(58.) The Stylo-glossus, which comes small and delicate from the root of the Styloid Procefs; expands as it goes towards the tongue, and whose office is to pull the tongue down into the mouth.

(59.) The Hyo-glossus, which I have represented as one single flat muscle, rising from nearly the whole length of the Os Hyoides *.

(60.) Is the Genio-glossus, so named from its rising from that point of the lower jaw bone (*o*), which is called the chin; its fibres go into the tongue in a radiated form, in every direction, capable of performing all kinds of motions, of lolling the tongue out, and also of retracting it again; whence this muscle has by way of pre-eminence

been

---

* From its arising in three fasciculi or distinct bundles, *viz.* one from the basis, one from the horn, and one from the Cartilage of the Os Hyoides, it has been called the Basio-chondro-cerato-glossus, or each fasciculus has occasionally been described, as a distinct muscle.

been named Mufculus Linguæ Pollychreftus. And *(r)* is the tongue itfelf, compofed chiefly of thefe mufcles, and covered with its membrane.

The Genio-hyoideus (38.) is a mufcle rifing from the fame point *(o)*, of the chin ; is
implanted into the Os Ilyoideus. This mufcle which rifes from the point of the chin
only, lies under the Mylo-hyoideus (37.) (*vide* Figure i.) which rifes from the whole
length of the jaw ; and thefe together pull the Os Hyoides, and of confequence the
throat upwards.

So that there is feen by thefe two drawings, firft, how the Mylo-hyoideus, (37.) figure i. and
the Genio-hyoideus, (38.) figure ii. pull the throat upwards. Secondly, how the Digaftric Mufcle (40.) and the three Styloid Mufcles, figure ii. pull the throat upwards
and backwards. Thirdly, how the Sterno-thyroidei, Sterno-hyoidei, and Omo-
hyoidei pull the throat downwards. And it is laftly very plain, that thefe at the fame
time that they are properly mufcles of the throat, are occafionally mufcles of the
lower jaw, the only ones indeed which pull it down ; little force is needed for this,
the jaw dropping almoft by its own weight ; but, as the motion muft be quick
and voluntary, it muft be done by mufcles ; and when the mufcles from the
Sternum fix the throat or pull it down, the Genio-hyoidei, Mylo-hyoidei and Biventer deprefs the jaw ; fo that the motions of the jaw and throat, or in other words,
the action of chewing and fwallowing have this confent, that they are partly performed by the fame common mufcles, fo that we cannot chew and fwallow at once ;
the jaw which moves in chewing the morfel, muft be fixed when it is to be fwal-
lowed ; and fo the motions for chewing and fwallowing alternately fucceed each
other.

PLATE

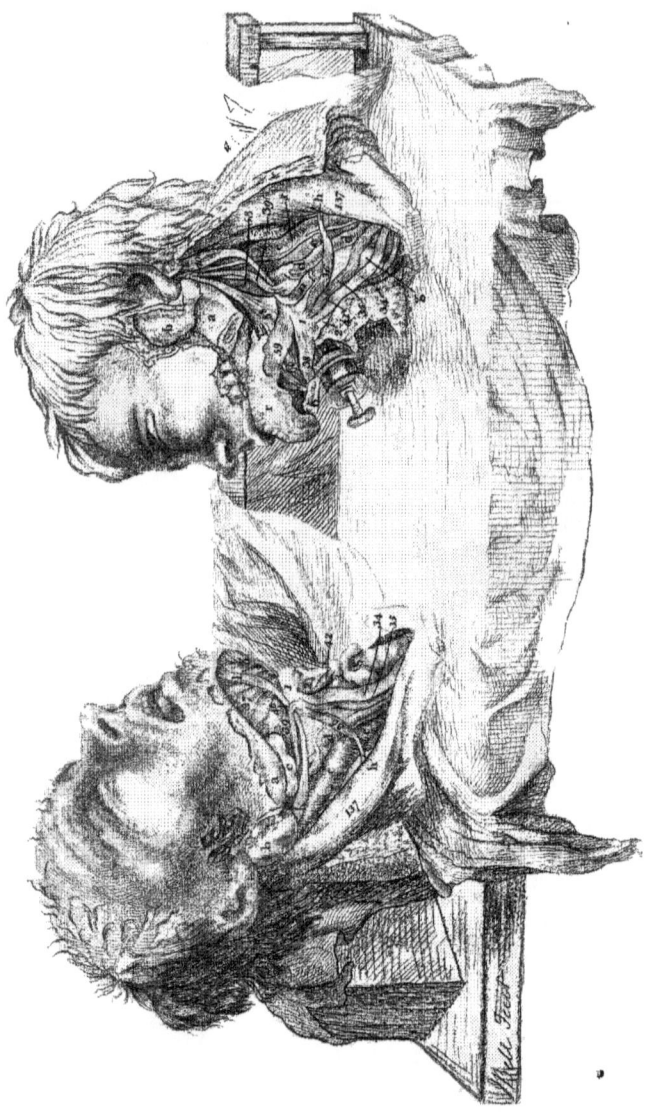
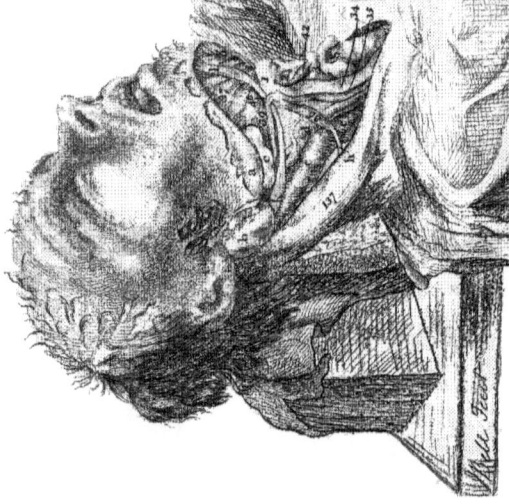

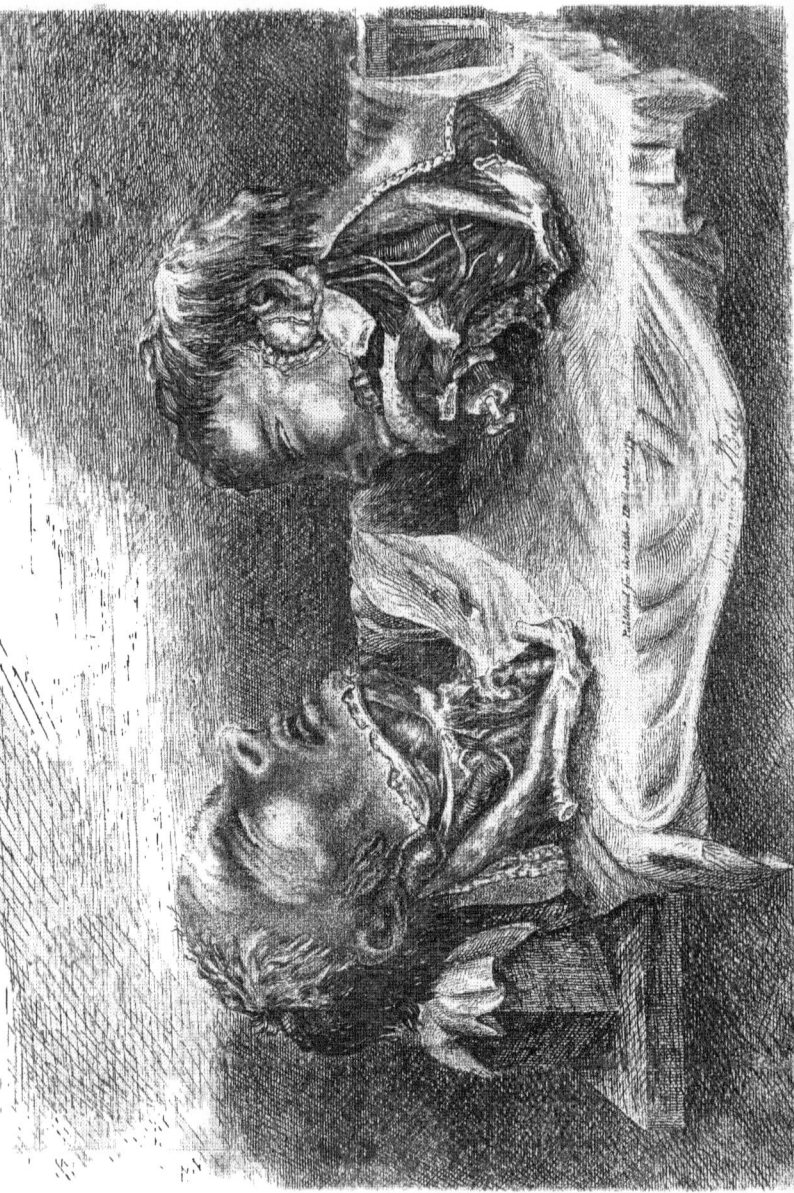

Pl. III.

MUSCLES.

P L A T E   IV.

This and the two following Plates explain the Text Book, from Page 232, to Page 285.

THIS plate explains thofe broad mufcles, which, belonging to the Scapula, lie flat upon the back, covering the whole of the trunk, and which are very remarkable in beautiful ftatues. The mufcles are chiefly the TRAPEZIUS, and the LATISSIMUS DORSI; and this drawing is not fo much of value as a piece of Anatomy, as in explaining to the ftudent the firft appearance of his diffection of the back; and by explaining the great mufcles of the Scapula, it marks a good beginning for the Anatomy of the arm.

THE TRAPEZIUS MUSCLE, (62) " is one of the moft beautiful mufcles of the body, of " a Lozenge-like form. Covers all the back and neck quite round to the fore-part of " the fhoulder; the two mufcles extend from the tip of the one fhoulder, to the " tip of the other, and from the nape of the neck quite down to the loins." The ftrong middle tendon by which the two mufcles of the oppofite fides are connected, is marked (a), the infertion into the Occiput is marked (b), and the infertion into the fpine of the Scapula, is marked (c).

" The LATISSIMUS DORSI, (70.) it is the broadeft not only of the back, but of the " whole body, covering all the lower parts of the back and loins." Its broad; flat,

and

and gliftening tendon is marked (*d*), the chief belly of the mufcle is marked with its number (70.); the place where its fibres crofs is marked (*e*), and it then runs under the arm into the deep fhadow, being implanted into the arm bone to pull the arm backwards.

The DELTOIDES (71.) next appears, the fkin being thrown down carelefsly, fo as to fhow where this mufcle rifes from the Spine of the Scapula; and efpecially its origin is feen; for it rifes from the Spine of the Scapula (*c*), and in part from that line of the Scapula into which the Trapezius Mufcle is inferted.

A fmall part of the TERES MAJOR, (76.) is feen in the fpace betwixt the Deltoides, and the Latiffimus Dorfi; a fmall part of the INFRA-SPINATUS, (74.) is feen lying upon the Scapula, under this (the back) part of the Deltoid; and alfo a fmall part of the Rhomboides, (65.) is feen under the edge of the Trapezius Mufcle. Upon the haunch, the upper part of the great Gluteus Mufcle (163.) is feen uncovered *of* by the fkin, which hangs like a fcroll over the edge of the table.

PLATE

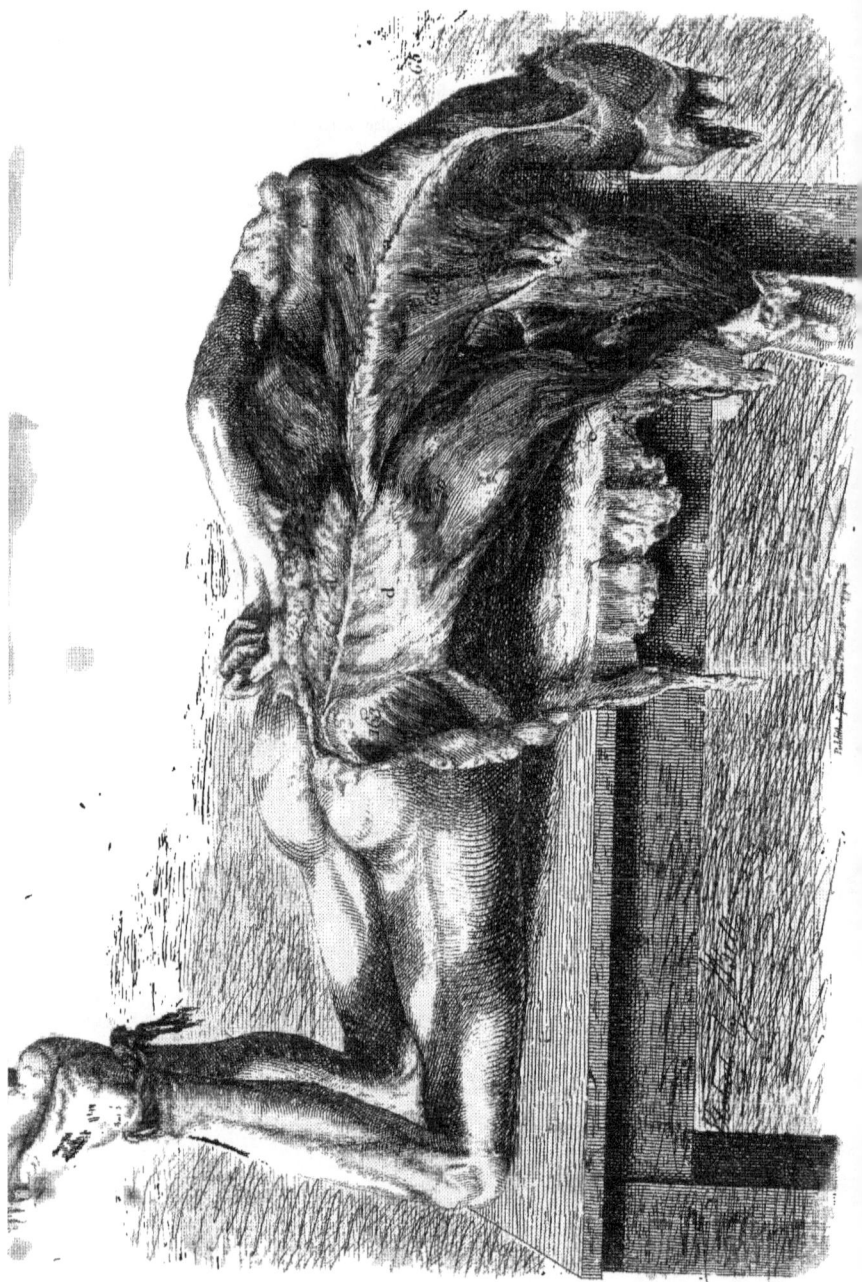

P L A T E   V.

This Plate with the IV. & VI. *explains the Text Book, from Page* 232, *to Page* 285.

THIS plate fhows the arm in that pofture into which it naturally falls, when thrown out upon the table, *viz.* ftanding upon the lower angle of the Scapula, the fhoulder joint raifed, and a little fupported, the elbow touching the table, the fore-arm lying flat along the table, the wrift raifed by the box of knives thruft under it, and the hand dropping over the box, fo as to touch the table again, with the knuckles.

FIGURE I. defcribes the outtermoft layer of Mufcles. Figure II. (a fuller diffection,) explains thofe which lie under, and contains every mufcle quite down to the bone. The two drawings are explained as one, fince they are indeed two drawings of the fame arm in one pofture; and the moft natural arrangement for this explanation is, 1. Of the mufcles lying on the Scapula, and moving the fhoulder bone. 2. Mufcles lying on the arm, and moving the Radius and Ulna, the two bones of the fore-arm, and 3. The mufcles which lie upon the fore-arm, and which move the wrift, and fingers, and thumb.

1. MUSCLES

I. MUSCLES LYING UPON THE SCAPULA.

There is feen here, the part of the SERRATUS MAJOR ANTICUS Mufcle, (66.) which lies upon the fore-part of the cheft, which goes backwards under the Scapula, betwixt it and the ribs; and which is implanted, as is feen here, into all the line of the Bafis of the Scapula, to pull it forwards. The place where the SUPRA-SPINATUS (73.) lies, above the Spine, is feen filled with its mufcle in the upper drawing, and the place of that mufcle is feen empty, and with only naked bone in the lower drawing.

The INFRA-SPINATUS, (74.) is feen both in the upper and in the lower drawing, covering all that part of the Scapula, which is below the Spine.

The TERES MINOR, (75.) is feen both in the upper and in the lower drawing, lying in its place not much diffeéted, and fo little feparated from the Infra-fpinatus (74.) that it looks rather like a particular fafciculus of that mufcle, as indeed it is; but though the Teres Minor is not in its flefhy belly eafily diftinguifhed from the Subfcapularis, yet it has its tendon very diftinét.

The TERES MAJOR, (76.) is neither like the Teres Minor, nor is it round as its name imports, but is a large, flat, and long mufcle which comes along with the Teres Minor, from the angle of the Scapula, and being here fully diffeéted, and hanging flabby, it is feen, that it twifts under the fhoulder bone, and is implanted, not like the Teres Minor, which goes into the knob on the outfide of the head of the fhoulder bone; but low down, and upon the fhaft of the bone, almoft as low as the infertion of the Deltoid Mufcle; fo that the fhoulder bone is embraced betwixt the two Teretes Mufcles, even in the natural condition of the parts; and in the aukward twiftings of a luxation, the head of the bone is often clofely embraced and ftrangled, as it were, betwixt the two Teretes mufcles, and not unfrequently under the fubfcapularis; an accident which makes the bone more difficult to reduce; but very often

the

the joint is not at all embraced by the mufcles, but is quite loofe and moveable, and its being eafily reduced, is rather perhaps to be confidered as a fign of the joint being much hurt and all thefe mufcles torn away.

(71.) Is the DELTOIDES, the laft mufcle which proceeds from the Scapula on this fide of the arm. It is feen here rifing from the Spine of the Scapula (a), from the tip of the Acromion Procefs (b), and alfo it has an origin from a part of the clavicle. It is feen here implanted in the arm bone at (d), about one third down. In the upper drawing it lies in its place; in the lower drawing it is cut up and turned backward, to fhow the head of the bone, and the infertion of the Teres Minor.

But there are ftill two other mufcles which rife from the Scapula, to be implanted into the arm bone, viz. the SUBSCAPULARIS, (77.) and the Coraco-brachialis, (72.) which are both feen in the next plate.

II. The Mufcles moving the fore-arm, and which lie' upon the arm, are the Triceps and Anconeus behind, and the Biceps and Brachialis Internus before.

The Triceps (80.) was once defcribed as three mufcles, but is now accounted as one mufcle, having three heads; (e) the firft, a long head, which rifes from the lower edge of the Scapula, near the Glenoid Cavity; and, coming down betwixt the Teres Major, and the Teres Minor Mufcles (75.) and (76.) meets the fecond head which is fhorter; for the fecond head of the Triceps (f), rifes from the fhoulder bone, a little below the head of the bone, and takes a long origin from almoft the whole length of the humerus. In thefe two drawings, the firft and fecond head only of the Triceps is feen; but in the next plate, the third or fhorteft head (g) of the Triceps is feen, coming rather from the inner fide of the bone, and lower down.

The ANCONEUS, (81.) or Mufcle of the Elbow, is a fmall mufcle not very eafily found nor underftood. It lies exactly upon that part of the elbow on which we reft in leaning upon the arm. It is feen in the upper drawing only, and is marked with its number (81).

P

(78.) The

(78.) The BICEPS, the Thick Mufcle of the fore part of the Arm, is feen in the upper
figure. But the middle of its belly only is feen; its heads lying under the Deltoid
Mufcle. The BRACHIALIS INTERNUS, (79.) which lies under the Biceps, is feen
in the uper drawing, but it is better feen in the lower drawing; and the manner of
its rifing from the fore part of the fhoulder-bone is tolerably well exprefled.
Neither of the heads of the Biceps can be feen in the upper drawing, becaufe
of the Deltoid Mufcle; but in the lower drawing, where the Deltoid is cut up
from the Scapula, and reclined backwards, the longer head of the Biceps is feen
raifed upon the blow-pipe, (b) which is paffed under it juft where the tendon is
coming out from the Capfule of the fhoulder joint; for this head of the Biceps is
a long and flender tendon, which comes from within the cavity of the fhoulder joint,
and goes down under the belly of the Deltoid Mufcle, being tendinous quite to the
middle of the arm.

The mufcles of the FORE ARM are arranged in my defcription of the Mufcles under
two claffes.

I. The Extenfors of the wrift, fingers, and thumb, which all keep the outer round
fide of the fore-arm, arifing chiefly from the outer Condyle.

II. The Flexors, or Benders of the wrift, fingers, and thumb, which lie all upon the
inner flat fide of the fore-arm, rifing in their turn, chiefly from the inner Condyle.
In thefe drawings the extenfors only can be feen; in the drawings of the next plate
all the flexors are feen.

To begin then with the Mufcles lying upon the upper or radial edge of the fore arm,
there is,

(92.) The SUPINATOR LONGUS RADII, which turns the palm of the hand up; for it rifes
from the fhoulder bone, above the elbow joint, and goes down the fore-arm with a
long flat tendon, which is marked (i) to be planted into the Radius at its fore-part.

(103.) The SUPINATOR RADII BREVIS, is a deeper Mufcle, and therefore it is feen
only

only in figure ii. where it is seen lying close upon the Inter-osseous Ligament, rising from the Ulna, going across to be inserted broad and fleshy into the Radius, and turning the Radius upon the Ulna, so as to throw the palm upwards.

The two next muscles keep also very exactly to the Radial edge of the arm; belong to the wrist; are the extensors of the wrist on the Radial side of the arm; and are named Extensores Carpi Longior et Brevior.

(93.) The EXTENSOR CARPI RADIALIS LONGIOR, rises from the arm bone just under the place of the Supinator Longus (92.); has a strong fleshy belly like it; and its long tendon accompanies the long tendon of the SUPINATOR, and is implanted near the root of the thumb, at (*k*), to bend the wrist back.

(94.) The EXTENSOR CARPI RADIALIS BREVIOR, rises also from the shoulder bone, but lower, and thence it is shorter; but it is in all other respects like the former; like it has a short thick fleshy belly; a long and slender tendon, running along the wrist, is implanted into the back of the hand, at the root of the fore-finger, at (*l*); and like the former it bends the wrist backwards.

These three muscles, the SUPINATOR, and the two extensors, form the chief flesh of the fore-arm just under the elbow joint, and the three bellies make three dimples and three curious swellings, which are drawn by the painter with great care, for they make the chief marks of the fore-arm; and the true drawing of the fore-arm (in its bendings and fore-shortenings, and especially in its strong exertions of pulling or grasping,) consists chiefly in the right placing of these three bellies, where they cover the joint; and it is the rising belly of the Supinator, which (in the drawing), joins the fore-arm rightly to the arm. These three muscles are seen lying in their places in the upper drawing, but flaccid. In the lower drawing, the SUPINATOR, (92.) is cut away, and the place, whence it was cut out from the arm-bone, is marked with its number (92.), while the long Extensor (93.) and the short Extensor (94.) are both left in their place; but they are much dissected, and allowed to hang

P 2

over by their own weight to the inner fide of the fore-arm, fo that in this lower
drawing their tendons are lefs perfectly feen.

(95.) The EXTENSOR CARPI ULNARIS is feen in the upper drawing diffected very
clean, lying loofe and flabby, but yet not feparated from the Ulna; whereas in
the lower drawing it is fo fully diffected, as to fall away from the Ulna, leaving
the bone at *(m)* naked.

And fo there remains of all the mufcles on this fide of the fore-arm, thofe only which
extend the fingers and thumb; and they are all feen, in the upper drawing, diffected,
but ftill in their places. In the lower arm they are all thrown loofe.

(96.) The EXTENSOR COMMUNIS DIGITORUM is feen in the upper drawing thick and
maffy; covering the other flender mufcles. This mufcle goes to all the fingers, by the
tendons *(n n)* which are feen on the back of the hand. In the upper figure the Extenfor Communis is in its place; in the lower drawing it is cut up, and thrown
out upon the table.

(97.) EXTENSOR DIGITI MINIMI vel Auricularis is feen only in the lower drawing, for
in the upper drawing it is covered by the Extenfor Communis. It is like a flip of
the Extenfor Communis, and confequently it is cut up here along with the
Extenfor Communis.

The flender tendons of the Extenfor Communis are marked *(n n.)* The flender tendon of
the Auricularis is marked *(o.)* But the fore finger alfo has a particular Extenfor,
which is named Indicator, and the thumb has three Extenfors, named 1ft, 2d, and 3d.

(98.) The EXTENSOR PRIMUS POLLICIS is the firft upon the edge of the arm, paffing obliquely over the Radius (99.) The EXTENSOR SECUNDUS is next to that; and the
EXTENSOR TERTIUS (100.) is next to that again. Thefe three Extenfors are feen fully
diffected in the lower drawing, hanging loofe, and their flender tendons diftinctly feen.
In the upper drawing they are lefs diffected; and the manner in which the three tendons crofs obliquely over the wrift, and the manner of their coming up to the thumb
touching the great joint of it, is well explained. It is feen here that thefe tendons are

bound

bound down by the Annular Ligament (*) ; and by raiſing the thumb ſtrongly in our own hand, we can compare it with this diſſeɛtion, for we ſee the ſtarting up of theſe tendons of the thumb, and we ſee at the ſame time the point diſtinɛtly marked at which the ring of the Annular Ligament holds them down.

The INDICATOR (101.) lies next to the Extenſor Tertius Pollicis ; it riſes from the Ul‐ na ; its ſlender tendon goes up to the fore-finger to extend it. This muſcle is ſeen on‐ ly in the lower drawing. In the upper drawing all the muſcles are in their na‐ tural places, the tendons being bound down by the Annular Ligament which is marked (*). It is a tendinous expanſion, thin, flat, and ribband-like, and the muſcles extending the fingers are ſeen through this tranſparent band. It is called the Annular, or Ring-like Ligament of the wriſt.

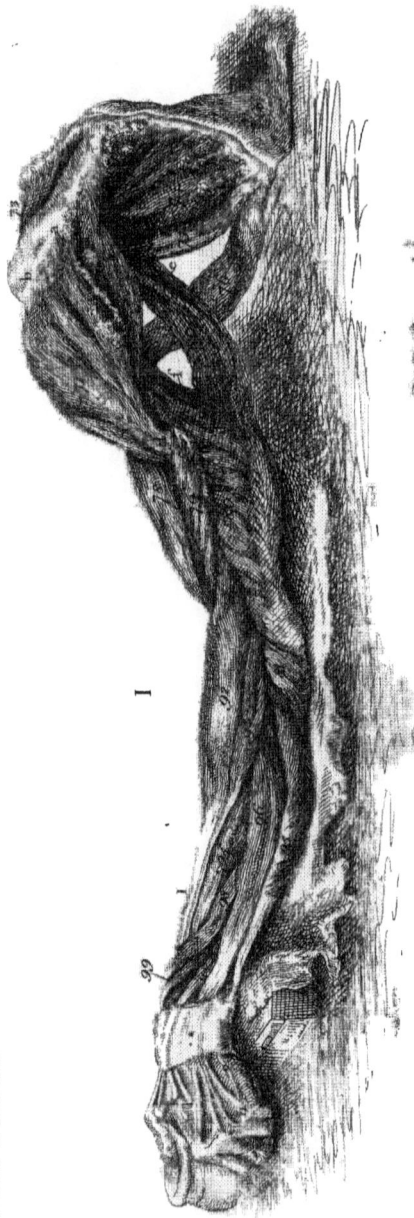

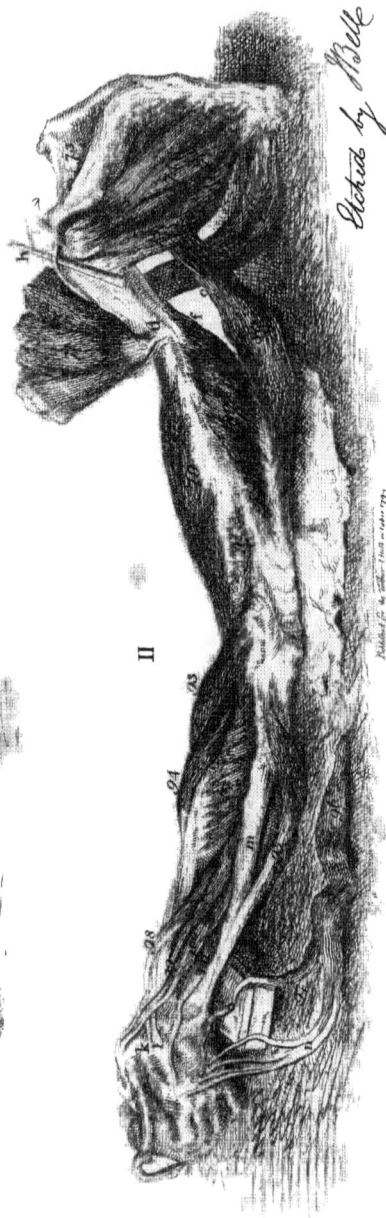

MUSCLES

PL.V.

I

II

Etched by Bell

PLATE VI.

This Plate explains the Text Book, from pag. 217, to page 220.

THIS plate explains all the flexor mufcles of the hand, wrift, and fingers, by a drawing taken when the arm was fet up for the figures of the laft plate, and confequently the poftures are exprefly the fame; and the parts, as the SCAPULA, the CLAVICLE, and the pofition of the fore-arm muft be eafily underftood.

THE Seratus Major Anticus (66.) is ftill feen hanging down from the bafis of the Scapula. Part of the Supra-fpinatus (73.) is feen above the Spine. ~~Below the Spine is feen the Infra-fpinatus.~~

The SUBSCAPULARIS (77.) is feen filling the whole of the hollow of the Scapula, lying der the Scapula, betwixt it and the ribs.

The TERES MAJOR (76.) is feen here alfo hanging down flaccid from the place, where it is implanted into the fhoulder bone.

That part of the DELTOIDES (71.) which rifes from the Clavicle (*a*) is feen here.

The BICEPS BRACHII (78.) is feen in the upper drawing with the belly marked (78), lying in its place. Its longer flender tendon which comes from within the fhoulder joint is marked (*b*). Its fhorter tendon which ftill is very long but thick and flefhy,

2   is

is feen marked (c), coming from under the Deltoid mufcle where it rifes from the Coracoid Procefs. Its flat tendon, which expands upon the fore-arm, and ftrengthens the general fafcia of the arm, is feen fpreading out over the mufcles at (d), and the ragged edges of the fafcia are feen lying out upon the mufcles, for the mufcles both above and below are diffected clean, while the fafcia of the arm is left only at (d), that the connection betwixt this fafcia and the Biceps tendon might be explained.

In the lower drawing the fhorter head of the Biceps (c) is feen cut away from the Cora- coid Procefs (e), and hung up by a ftring. The longer head (b) is pulled upwards by a ftring, that it may be feen how it comes from under the clavicle, where it rifes within the fhoulder joint. The Coracoid Procefs whence the fhorter head arifes is marked (e), and it is feen that there are three points of mufcles fticking to the apex of the procefs; for the little pectoral mufcle (67.) is implanted into it; and the CORACO-BRACHIALIS (72.) and this fhorter head of the Biceps rife from it.

The BRACHIALIS INTERNUS (79.) is feen in both arms, lying under the belly of the Bi- ceps, and rifing from the bone.

The CORACO-BRACHIALIS (72.) is feen in both the drawings. In the upper drawing it is touched by the fhort head of the Biceps, which makes it lefs diftinct. In the low- er drawing the fhort head of the Biceps is tucked up. The Coraco-brachialis is fully diffected, and is left flaccid and hanging away from the arm bone; and its ori- gin from the Coracoid Procefs (e), and its infertion into the middle of the fhoul- der bone at (g) are both well feen.

Over the middle of the bending of the Coraco-brachialis there is feen the remains of a flat and broad tendon, (69.) fticking to the arm bone, which is the cut tendon of the great pectoral mufcle, which is implanted thus low upon the Os Humeri, to give it the advantage of a lever in pulling the fhoulder bone inwards. I have ufed the mark (69.) of the pectoral mufcle to point out its tendon.

The TRICEPS (80.) is alfo well feen, efpecially two of its heads, viz. the longeft head (f,) and the fhorteft head (g), while the head which is of a middle length lies upon the back part of the bone, and cannot be feen in this view.

The

The mufcles of the FORE-ARM, *i. e.* all the Flexors of the hand, fingers, and thumb, are fhown here; in the upper drawing, they are in their natural pofition, in the lower drawing, they are feparated for demonftration, and fome of them are hung out.

In the upper drawing, the mufcles of the fore-arm are few and fimple, lying regularly in their places; and fo are eafily underftood.

One mufcle belonging to the outfide of the arm is feen here, *viz.* the SUPINATOR RADII LONGUS, (92.) the belly of which is feen lying upon the Radial edge of the arm, above the elbow; the next to that is the PRONATOR TERES, (82.) It rifes at (*b*), from the internal Condyle; is implanted into the Radius at (*i*), and turns the hand prone, (*i. e.*) flat down. It is called Pronator Teres, becaufe it has a round flefhy belly, very oppofite in fhape to the Pronator Quadratus; for the PRONATOR QUADRATUS, (91.) which is feen in the lower drawing is of a fquare form, lying flat upon the Inter-offeous Membrane, rifing from the Ulna, implanted into the Radius, and having only one direct office, *viz.* that of turning the Radius.

The next mufcle to the Pronator Teres, is the FLEXOR CARPI RADIALIS, (85.) or the bender of the wrift, on the fide of the Radius. Its head is covered in part by the expanding tendon of the biceps at (*d*); then the reft of the mufcle is naked; and its long tendon is feen as it goes along the Radial edge of the fore-arm marked (*k*).

The PALMARIS LONGUS, (83.) is a long, flender, and delicate mufcle; it is merely a bender of the wrift; and comes by a fmall head from the inner Condyle of the Humerus, and its fmall tendon runs down the middle of the arm till it touches the Anular Ligament of the wrift, to be implanted into it. This Anular Ligament I have marked (*); but though it has the fame mark with the Anular Ligament on the outfide of the arm, it is not a continuation of the fame Ligament, nor is it like it; but is a fhort, thick, and very ftrong ligament paffing acrofs from the Pifiform, to the Scaphoid bone of the Carpus. It is fhorter and ftronger than the Anular Ligament of the outfide; it has a firmer origin from two particular bones,

Q   and

and has a deeper arch under it: for the tendons which it binds down are very numerous, and connected with much stronger muscles than those on the back of the hand.

The FLEXOR CARPI ULNARIS, (86.) lies along the ulnar edge of the arm; is a penniform or feather-like muscle, very fleshy; rises from the inner Condyle along with the Palmaris Longus, (83.) and is implanted by a strong round tendon into the projecting Pisiform Bone.

The FLEXOR DIGITORUM SUBLIMIS, (87.) is a very large thick bellied muscle. It is called Sublimis, because it is the outtermost of the two flexor muscles. It is seen here lying in its place, thick and fleshy in its belly; its tendons passing under the arch of the Anular Ligament, appearing in the palm of the hand, to go to all the fingers; there are four distinct tendons, which are here supported upon a blow-pipe marked (m); and the place of the Flexor Profundus, which lies under, it is seen at (88.)

In the lower drawing, the muscles of the fore-arm are seen much freer and better.

The PRONATOR TERES (82.) is seen in its place, thick, round, and fleshy.

The PALMARIS LONGUS, (83.) is thrown out upon the table; by which it is seen how short and delicate its muscular belly is; how long, slender, and delicate its tendon (n), from which it has got its name. And the Palmar Apponeurosis, or tendinous web, (l), which covers the palm of the hand, and which like the palm is of a triangular form, is here cut up and left connected with its tendon.

The UPPER Flexor of the fingers, or FLEXOR SUBLIMIS, (87.) is supported by a ligature, so as to draw its four tendons nearly into a straight line, showing how they are split near the fingers, whence this muscle is often named PERFORATUS.

The deep Flexor, FLEXOR PROFUNDUS, (88.) is left at its origin. Its belly is raised and drawn out a little, and held extended by a pin; and the three tendons of this muscle are seen going through the loops, or splits of the tendon of the last muscle, whence this one is named Musculus Perforans.

The

These tendons of the Perforans and Perforatus are also well seen in the uppermost figure, where the perforating tendons are raised over the blowpipe (*o*), and the perforated tendons are also supported upon another blowpipe (*m*).

The muscle marked (88 *) which seems to go with a particular tendon towards the fore-finger, as if it were a particular Flexor for the fore-finger, is merely that head of the general Flexor which goes to the fore-finger, it is a part of the Flexor Profundus; and this particular appearance is produced merely by dissecting this belly a little too high up; for this muscle, and the Flexor Sublimis also, are divided or diviseable into four distinct bellies, for each of the four distinct fingers which they serve.

The FLEXOR LONGUS POLLICIS, (90.) is a large and strong muscle for bending the last joint of the thumb; its tendon is seen going in under the two short muscles of the thumb, and is seen again at (*q*) escaping from betwixt the short Flexors, and going forwards to the point of the thumb.

The PRONATOR QUADRATUS, (91.) is seen lying flat upon the Interosseous Membrane which is marked (*p*).

The muscles of the HAND are not fully explained, but yet the chief muscles are seen.

The ABDUCTOR BREVIS POLLICIS, (103.) is seen in the upper drawing rising from the outside of the Annular Ligament.

The FLEXOR BREVIS POLLICIS, (105) is seen rising also from the Annular Ligament. Another head rises deeper in the hand, but is not seen here, there is seen only the tendon of the long Flexor, passing betwixt these two heads of the short Flexor.

The OPPONENS POLLICIS, (104.) cannot be seen here, because it does not move any of the joints of the thumb. It belongs only to the Metacarpal Bone of the thumb; and of course it lies under these two.

The ADDUCTOR POLLICIS, (106.) or, that which carries the thumb towards the fore-finger, is also seen here; but so much under shadow, that it is not to be dis-tinguished from the ABDUCTOR INDICIS, (110.) For the Adductor Pollicis and

Q 2   Abductor

Abductor Indicis lie clofe upon each other, and are of the fame flat and triangular fhape.

The mufcles of the little finger are, the Abductor and the Flexor Minimi Digiti ;
but it is the ABDUCTOR MINIMI DIGITI (107.) only that is feen here, lying on
the edge of the palm, under the little finger ; which we feel acting, when we
fpread wide the little finger, or when taken with that flight cramp which we often
feel upon the lower edge of the palm.

PLATE

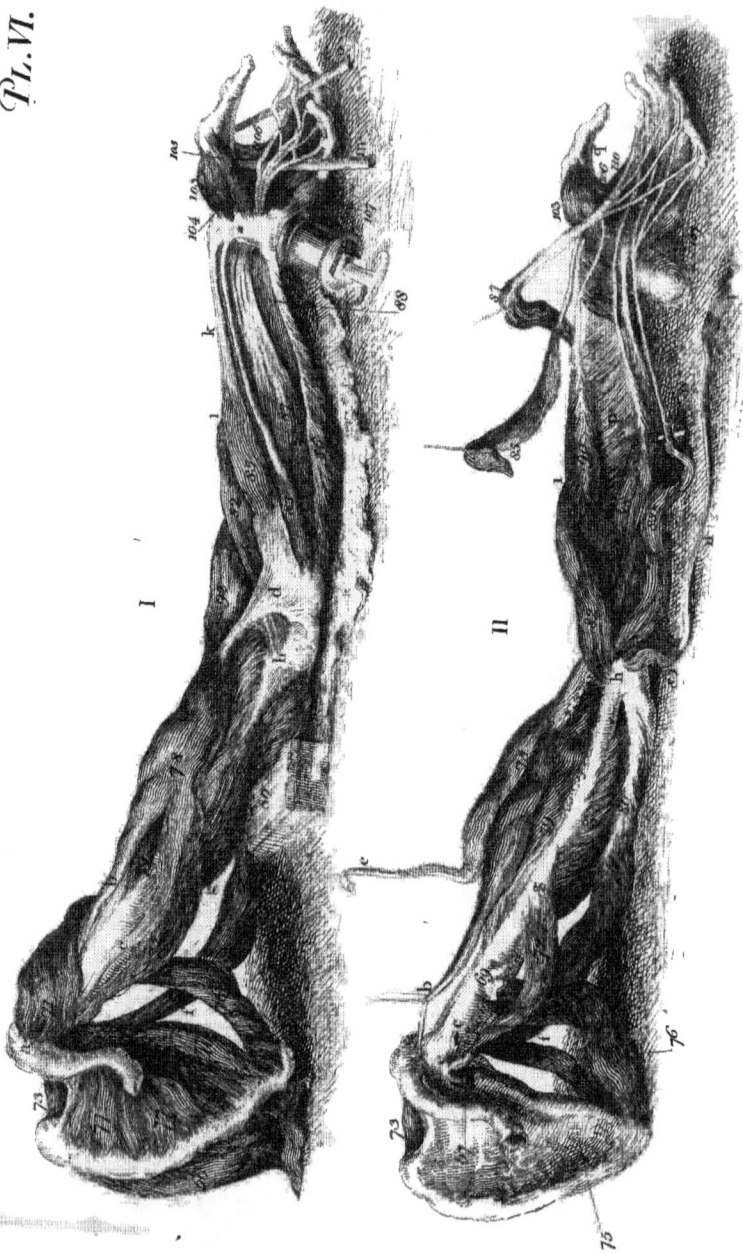

MUSCLES

Pl. VI.

I

II

Pallas for the anat. 1794

P L A T E   VII.

This Plate explains the Text Book, from Page 235, to Page 310.

THIS plate reprefents the Trunk of the body in various drawings; explaining thofe mufcles of the Scapula, which lie flat under the Trapezii Mufcles;—alfo the ferrated mufcles, which raife or deprefs the ribs in breathing; the LONGISSIMUS DORSI, and Sacro-Lumbalis, the chief mufcles which fupport the Spine; and it alfo explains the Intercoftal Mufcles; the Levators of the ribs; the leffer mufcles of the neck and Spine; and the RECTI CAPITIS, the fmall nodding mufcles of the head.

IT explains a fet of mufcles, which are found in the book from page 235, to page 310. From page 235 of the book, forwards, are explained the chief mufcles of the Scapula; as the Levator Scapulæ, the Rhomboid Mufcles, and the Serratus Anticus; and thefe three are the chief outermoft mufcles in the diffection reprefented in figures i. and ii.

The LEVATOR SCAPULÆ, (63.) is feen in Figure I. on both fides, rifing from the Tranfverfe Proceffes of the upper Vertebræ of the neck, and going downwards to be implanted into the upper corner of the Scapula, whence it is named Mufculus Angularis Scapulæ.

The RHOMBOID mufcles, (64, and 65.) are two flat mufcles which come with a thin

2   flat

flat tendon from the Spines of the neck and back, and are implanted quite fleſhy, but ſtill thin and flat, into the whole length of the baſis of the Scapula. The diviſion betwixt the cervical portion of this muſcle, (64.) which is the Rhomboides Minor, and the larger portion coming from the Spines of the back, and which is named Rhomboides Major, (65.) is very ſlight.

Part of the Infra Spinatus, (74.) is ſeen here; the Deltoides, (71.) is alſo ſeen; the Serratus Major Anticus, (66.) or great muſcle for moving the Scapula forwards, is ſeen lying upon the ſide of the cheſt, riſing from the ribs to paſs under the Scapula, where it is implanted into the whole length of the Baſis of the Scapula, exactly oppoſite to the inſertion of the Rhomboides. But in Figure II. the Serratus Major Anticus is repreſented again lying under the Scapula; and the Scapula, to ſhow it, is cut almoſt away from the trunk, and is thrown out into a very unnatural poſition, and the confluence of the ſeparate heads or Serræ by which this muſcle riſes from each of the ribs is indiſtinctly marked.

Thus the Serratus Anticus is ſeen to be a muſcle belonging to the Scapula; but the Serrati Postici, (113. 114.) are muſcles of the ribs belonging chiefly to reſpiration, and they are ſeen in Figure I. and theſe muſcles of the ribs are explained in the book from page 285, to page 290. The upper Serrated muſcle lies flat under the Rhomboides; the lower Serrated muſcle lies in like manner flat under the Latiſſimus Dorſi muſcle; but they cover the Longissimus Dorſi and Sacro-lumbalis muſcles, the lower Serratus covering their fleſhy bellies, and the uppermoſt covering their tendons.

The Serratus Superior Posticus (113.) is ſeen lying flat upon the ſide of the neck; on the right ſide the Rhomboides covers it; on the left ſide it is ſeen naked. It begins by a neat flat ſhining tendon, reſplendent like the colours of a fiſh turning in the water; and this flat tendon (which is exactly like the flat tendon of the Rhomboid muſcle) comes from the three lower Spines of the neck, and divides into three neat ſmall fleſhy heads which are marked (a a), and theſe are implanted into three

of

of the ribs ; and by raising three ribs it is plain that they muſt raiſe the whole cheſt.

The SERRATUS INFERIOR POSTICUS (114.) is the exact antagoniſt of this, and exactly like it in all reſpects, only that it goes obliquely from below upwards, to pull the ribs down. It ariſes by a ſilvery ſhining tendon like the upper one ; the tendon is very ſtrong, but thinner than a ſheet of paper. It ends in three heads, which are thin flat ſlips of fleſh, inſerted into the three or four lower ribs a little beyond their angles.

The LEVATORES COSTARUM, (115.) are concealed by theſe muſcles, but are ſeen in the next diſſection, Figure II. where they are ſeen to be in number twelve pairs correſponding with the number of the ribs. The nine uppermoſt are ſeen to be ſhort ; the three lower pairs are ſeen to paſs one rib, and to take hold on the rib below. Whence they are named LEVATORES COSTARUM LONGIORES.

The Levatores Coſtarum are theſe twelve diſtinct muſcles, riſing from the tranſverſe proceſs of each vertebra, and going down to lay hold upon each rib ; and ſo they lie flat upon the outſide of the ribs, and keep cloſe to the Spine, and are ſhort. But there are beſides regular plans of fibres lying in the interſtices of the ribs, which go from the edge of one rib to the edge of another, and fill up the ſpace betwixt the ribs and hence are named INTERCOSTALS. The internal intercoſtals exactly reſemble the external intercoſtals. The external intercoſtals only can be ſeen here, and they are ſeen beſt in the left ſide of figure ii. marked (116.) the three lower internal intercoſtal muſcles lying upon the three lower ribs are longer than the others, juſt as the lower Levators are longer; but it is not ſo in the outer layer of intercoſtals which (except in a few ſtraggling fibres) are all of equal length.

The muſcles which raiſe the trunk from the ſtooping poſture, and eſpecially the QUADRATUS LUMBORUM, SACRO-LUMBALIS, LONGISSIMUS DORSI, TRANSVERSALIS COLLI, and CERVICALIS, are explained from page 297, to page 301. and they are all pretty diſtinctly marked in figures i. and ii.

In FIGURE I. the LONGISSIMUS DORSI (126.) and the Sacro Lumbalis (127.) are ſeen only in the middle of the back ; for they are covered by the Rhomboid and Serratus

ſuperior

superior mufcles above, and in the fame way by the Serratus inferior Pofticus below; but in figure ii. the three great mufcles of the Spine, *viz.* the QUADRATUS
LUMBORUM (125.) the LONGISSIMUS DORSI (126.) and the Sacro-Lumbalis (127.)
are feen quite uncovered, and in their whole length; for their tendinous origin in
the loins at (*b*), their middle bellies at (126, 127.) and their long tendinous infertions at (*c*), are all diftinctly feen; and alfo their connection with the CERVICALIS
DESCENDENS (128.) is explained.

The QUADRATUS LUMBORUM, (125.) which is cut away on the right fide, is feen diftinctly on the left fide, arifing big and flefhy from the Spine of the Ilium, and inferted partly into the tranfverfe procelfes of the loins, but chiefly into the loweft rib.

The common tendon of the Longiffimus Dorfi, and of the Sacro-Lumbalis, is feen at
(*b*); it is a firm, thick, and ftrong origin, which is thus entirely tendinous without,
but flefhy within; it rifes from the SACRUM, ILIUM, and tranfverfe procelfes of
the Vertebræ, and fills up all the hollow upon both fides of the Spine.

The belly of the SACRO-LUMBALIS (127.) parts from the belly of the LONGISSIMUS
DORSI, (126.) at the top of the loins, nearly oppofite to the loweft rib.

The Longiffimus Dorfi keeps clofer by the Spine, and is inferted by a double row of
tendinous feet; but they lie fo under its own belly, and under the belly of the Sacro-Lumbalis, that they are hidden from the view. The tendinous feet of the SACRO-
LUMBALIS are well feen, fpreading out wider from the Spine and attaching themfelves
to the ribs; and thefe tendons marked (*c c*) are feen in figure i. lying flat and regular, each in its right place; but in figure ii. they are more diffected, are torn up a little from the flat furface of the ribs, and hang fomewhat loofe and flaccid. On the
right fide of the neck is feen the CERVICALIS DESCENDENS, (128.) rifing from the
tranfverfe procelfes of the neck, going down to be implanted tendinous into the back,
(*i. e.*) into the ribs. The Cervicalis is inferted under the upper tendons of the
Sacro-Lumbalis, and the Longiffimus Dorfi, on the other hand, is feen to fend a delicate flip of tendon up into it; fo that the Cervicalis feems equally connected with
                                                                              both

both of thefe mufcles, but it is rather more beholden to the Longiffimus Dorfi, for this flip; while the accident of the Cervicalis rifing under the tendinous feet of the Sacro-Lumbalis makes hardly any connection.

On the left fide again there is feen, the TRANSVERSALIS COLLI (129.); which rifing from the Tranfverfe Proceffes of the back, afcends towards the Tranfverfe Pro-ceffes of the neck; it is rather ftrong and flefhy, has little connection with any other mufcle; the Cervicalis Defcendens lies under it, while this the Tranfverfalis is in its turn covered by the Splenius and Complexus *.

R   The

* There are three flender mufcles in the neck, which are in danger of being confounded, viz. the TRACHELO-MASTOIDEUS, the TRANSVERSALIS CERVICIS, and the CERVICALIS DESCENDENS. It is impoffible to give a perfect drawing on fo fmall a fcale, nor indeed is it poffible by any drawing, to reprefent them fo that they fhall be eafily found, and diftinguifhed; perhaps they will beft be found by following this order of diffection. 1. The Trapezius and the Rhomboides, the two large flat external mufcles belonging to the Scapula, are to be cut away; and then the Serratus Superior where it covers the lower part of the Complexus is to be raifed. 2. The Splenius and Complexus are to be diffected and laid afide; and 3. the Trachelo-maftoideus, and the two other mufcles come into view. Of thefe, FIRST, there lies immediately under the Complexus the Trachelo-maftoideus, large and flefhy, rifing from the Tranfverfe Proceffes in the back and lower part of the neck, by tendinous and flefhy feet, and going obliquely upwards and outwards till it is implanted flefhy into the Maftoid Procefs; and though it is more flefhy than the two mufcles which come next, it ftill is fo much a mix-ture of tendon and flefh, as to be named the Complexus Minor.—SECONDLY, There is the TRANSVER-SALIS CERVICIS, which lies immediately under the Trachelo-maftoideus, keeps clofe to the Spine, i. e. lies in the hollow by the fide of the Spinous Proceffes. It rifes from the Tranfverfe Proceffes of the back to be implanted in the Tranfverfe Proceffes of the neck; is immediately covered by the Trachelo-Maftoideus; and covers in part the Cervicalis Defcendens.—THIRDLY, there is the CER-VICALIS DESCENDENS, which lies more to one fide than the Tranfverfalis Cervicis; it therefore lies more properly under the Trachelo-Maftoideus; its feet or tendinous origins begin from the tips of the Tranfverfe Proceffes of the neck, juft where the feet or fmall tendons of the Levator Scapulæ begin; it is very flender and is a confufed mixture of tendon and flefh, being chiefly ten-dinous, though it is flefhy in part. It is neceffary to give this warning, that not even the largeft drawing can make this piece of diffection perfectly eafy; perhaps it may be the eafier for this de-fcription and arrangement.

The rising slip of the Longissimus Dorsi has led to this explanation of the Transversalis, and of the Cervicalis Descendens; but naturally before these, there should have been explained the two larger muscles which cover them, viz. the Splenius and Complexus, which are best seen in figures i. and iii. In figure i. are seen, the Splenii (118.) straight and flat, lying along the side of the neck, like the legs of the letter V. and in the interstice or place of their forking, is seen the chief belly of the Complexus, (119.) where it is implanted into the Occiput, lying under the Splenii. In figure iii. the Splenii are cut away, the Complexus only is seen, the chief belly of the Complexus where it is implanted into the Os Occipitis is marked with its proper number (119.); while its feet (partly tendinous and partly fleshy), by which it rises from the Transverse Processes of the neck and back, are marked (e e).

The muscles belonging exclusively to the Spine, are next seen in figure iii. for the chief of them are these two, First, the Spinalis Dorsi, (131.) or long muscle belonging to the Spinous Processes of the back. It runs along the whole back from spine to spine; it is very slender and almost entirely tendinous, and is marked with its number, (131.) Secondly, the Multifidus Spinæ, (133.) which is a confused mixture of tendon and flesh, but thick and massy enough to fill all the hollow over the Oblique Processes of the Vertebræ, and betwixt the Spinous and Transverse Processes.

Three of the four small muscles which perform the quick turning and nodding motions of the head, are explained upon the head, figure iv. where the two small muscles called Recti Capitis are seen dissected fairly, and laid over a blow-pipe; and here it will be observed that the two Recti Minores (121.) are smaller, and lie deeper betwixt the Atlas and the Scull; that the Rectus Major (122.) is not, as its name implies, a straight muscle, but is truely oblique. One of the Oblique muscles is also shown here, for there are two oblique muscles, somewhat like the Recti or straight ones. The Oblique Muscle (123.) which is here shown, is the

2   -   Obliquus

Obliquus Superior, which rifes from the Tranfverfe Procefs of the Atlas, to be inferted into the Occiput. The Obliquus inferior, which rifes from the Dentatus to be fixed into the Atlas is here cut away, for only the Atlas is left in this drawing.

yet the Rectus Major arises from the spine of the Dentatus

R 2 PLATE

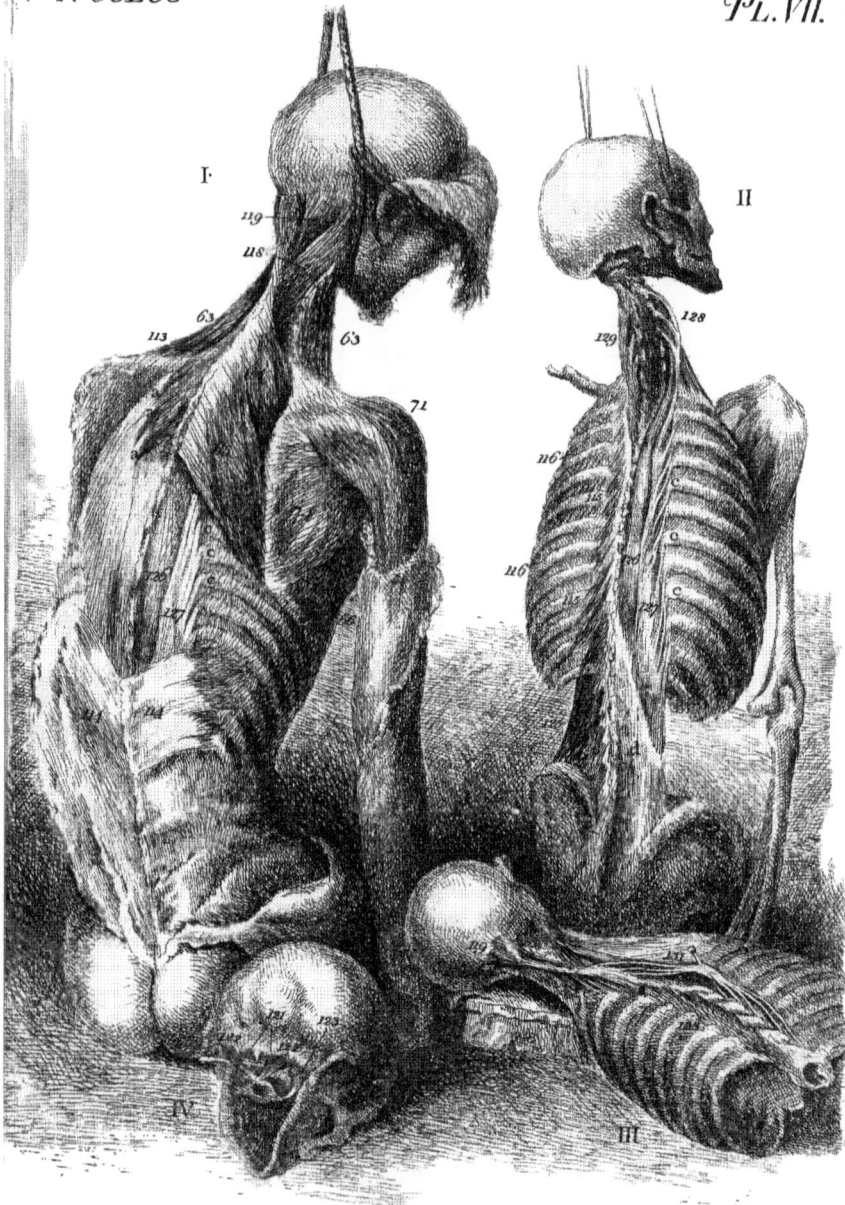

I.

II.

III.

IV.

The drawings and plans which are numbered, VIII. IX. X. & XI. explain chapter vi. and vii. of the book, contain-
ing the Abdominal Muscles, the Diaphragm, and the muscles of the Perinæum.
Plate VIII. gives a general view of the Abdominal Muscles, as they are first laid open. Plate IX. gives a second dissec-
tion of the Abdominal Muscles, showing the successive layers of the great Muscles which cover the Abdomen. Plate X.
explains the general appearance of the Diaphragm, and its relation to the body. Plate XI. explains by plans and
drawings, the Diaphragm and the muscles of the parts of generation.

P L A T E   VIII.

EXPLAINS the first dissection of the Abdominal Muscles in a lateral view;
and the chief intention of the drawing is, to show the general appearance of the belly when uncovered of its skin; to show the great size of
the Musculus Obliquus Externus, " and how it covers all the side with
" its fleshy belly, and all the fore-part of the Abdomen with its thin
" expanded tendon;" to explain the two great lines or marks, the
Linea Alba, and Linea Semi-lunaris, and to show the ring of the Abdominal Muscles, and the ligament of the thigh in their true shapes, with
the exit of the great arteries of the thigh, and the passage of the Spermatic Cord.

THE description then of these few parts needs not be tedious.

First, the great belly of the EXTERNAL OBLIQUE Muscle of the ABDOMEN is marked
with its proper number (143.); and it is seen here how it covers the side, how it
lies out upon the fore-part of the Thorax, and how it rises from the ribs by indigita-
tions,

tious, which are marked fo dark that they can be underflood only by the indigita-
tions (a a a) of the Serratus Major Anticus Mufcle, in the interftices of which
they rife.

The belly of this mufcle covers only the fide, ftops fuddenly at (b b), which reprefent
the flat tendon, the fibres of which go obliquely from above downwards and inwards, where it is named OBLIQUUS DESCENDENS. The letters (c c c) fhow the
line which is called LINEA SEMI-LUNARIS; and the letters are fo placed, as alfo
to point out the interfections or tendinous lines which divide the Recti, or ftraight
mufcles of the Abdomen, into four or five diftinct bellies; and confequently the
letters (c c c) alfo mark the feveral bellies of the Rectus, fhining through the thin
expanded tendon of the External Oblique.

(*) Marks the head of the Rectus Mufcle, where it rifes from the border of the
Thorax, touching the PECTORAL MUSCLE (69.), and at the place of this mark (*),
the mufcle is uncovered of its fheath; this mark ferves alfo another ufe, for it is
repeated again below near the navel, fo that thefe two marks fhow the whole
length of the LINEA ALBA, or white line, which is feen running down all the center
of the belly from the Sternum quite to the Pubis, paffing through the navel, and
formed by the meeting of the tendons of all the mufcles. And it is perhaps
worth notice, that the fmall holes marked very dark, which are neat, fmall, and
round, and which appear in every diffection, like Oilet Holes, and are efpecially frequent over the furfaces of the Recti Mufcles, are juft the openings by
which the great Cutaneous Veins of the Abdomen pierce the flat tendon of the
External Oblique Mufcle, to get to the bellies of the Mufcles which lie under it, or
rather to come back from them, returning chiefly the blood of the Epigaftric
Artery†.

The

† I queftion whether it be not truely a wound of one of thefe large veins, (and they are greatly
dilated in dropfy of the belly), which occafions that kind of bleeding, which fo often happens in
tapping the belly.

The tendency of the Oblique fibres of the Abdominal Muscle to split is easily seen, and the manner of its spliting to form the RING of the ABDOMINAL MUSCLES is faithfully reprefented, where (*d*) marks the lower pillar of the ring ; (*e*) the upper pillar of the ring ; and it is plain that (*d*) while it forms the lower pillar of the ring, is at the fame time the Ligament of the thigh. (*f*) Marks the Spermatic Cord coming through the opening of the ring ; (*g*) marks the femoral Artery coming from under Paupart's Ligament, or the Ligament of the thigh. Whence it will be underftood how Bubonocele or Hernia of the Groin, following the courfe of the Spermatic Cord, will proceed obliquely inwards, and muft (in attempting to reduce it), be pufhed from within outwards : and how a femoral Hernia will by coming out from under the femoral Ligament, be lodged fairly in the thigh, far from the Groin; lying very deep, apt to be concealed from the Surgeon; and how by following the courfe of the great veffels of the thigh, the Femoral Hernia will proceed from within obliquely outwards, fo that, in attempting to reduce this Hernia, we muft pufh from without obliquely inwards.

PLATE

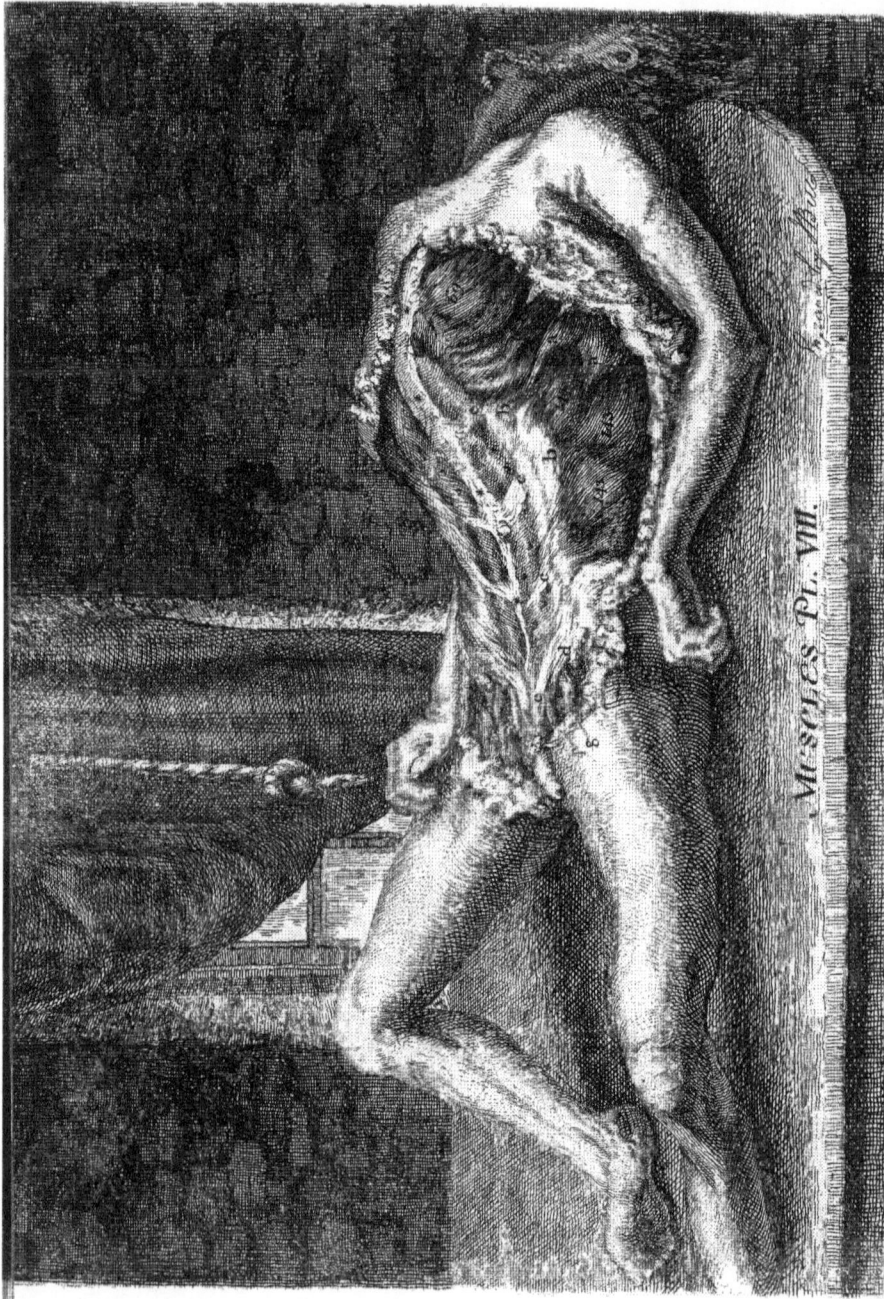

P L A T E   IX.

This Plate along with the former explains the Text Book, from page 311, to page 323.

EXPLAINS the fecond diffection of the belly; where the mufcles being
cut and thrown out upon the thighs, may feem irregular and confufed,
though it is truly the natural order and true appearance of the diffection. The view is not fore-fhortened enough to make a pleafant drawing, becaufe it was neceffary to look from a high point, as in feeing
a diffection from the feats of a Theatre, in order to have a full view of
all the belly, from the Pubis to the Sternum.

1. The EXTERNAL OBLIQUE MUSCLE, (143.) is entirely cut away, and no part of it
remains on either fide.

2. The INTERNAL OBLIQUE MUSCLE (144.) is feen on both fides; on the left fide of the
body it is cut up from its infertion, and is thrown down upon the thigh, fhowing
chiefly how thick and ftrong its flefhy belly is; but on the right fide of the body it
is left in its place, where the obliquity of its fibres is well feen, and where the
chief points of the defcription are fulfilled in the drawing, *viz.* that the chief
belly of the Obliquus Internus is at the Iliac Spine, that the central fibres only are
direct, going acrofs the Abdomen to the Linea Alba; and that the higher fibres

S   afcend

afcend towards the Sternum, while the lower ones go obliquely downwards to the
Pubis. This is the mufcle which gives that mufcular covering of the Spermatic
Cord, ftrong in animals, though weak in man, which is named Cremafter. The
tefticle of the right fide is torn up from the Scrotum, and thrown out upon the
thigh, that the conneftion of the Spermatic Cord with this the Internal Oblique
Mufcle, might be feen; and although it could not be diftinftly expreffed in fo
fmall a figure, without exaggerating and departing from the true drawing, yet there
is a conical form of the Spermatic Cord at its upper end, which fhows where the
Cremafter Mufcle joins it.

;. The TRANSVERSALIS ABDOMINIS, (145.) is feen on the left fide. It looks at firft fight
much like the Internal Oblique, but it is to be remembered, that the Internal Oblique of this fide (144.) is thrown down over the thigh. The TRANSVERSE
fends all its fibres direftly acrofs the Abdomen; and it is feen to belong to the
inner furface of the Thorax, as much as the External Oblique Mufcle belongs to.
the outer furface of it. (a a) Reprefent the place where the flefh of this mufcle
ends, and the tendon begins; and the tendon at this point is ftrongly attached to
the tendon of the inner Oblique Mufcle. The letters (a a) mark the edge where the
two thin tendons adhere to form the fheath for the RECTUS MUSCLE; the letter (b) is
placed in the fheath itfelf; the fheath is feen again on the left fide empty, and marked
(b b); with the bowels of the Abdomen fhinning through the back part of the
fheath, which though very denfe and ftrong, is yet thin and almoft tranfparent.
But at the lower part (c), it is lefs perfeft, or rather is wanting; the thinner
membrane of the Peritoneum only being found there.

4. The RECTUS ABDOMINIS, (146.) of the left fide remains in its place; it is diffefted.
on its fore-part, fo as to fhow the tendinous interfeftions (d d), where the fore-
part of the fheath adheres; but at the back of the fheath, (i. e.) at (b) there are
no fuch adhefions, and though the Reftus is fo attached at the fore-part, as to be
                                                                                    very

very difficultly diffected; it lies at its back part fo loofely, that it is eafily turned out of its fheath with the point of the finger, or the handle of the diffecting knife.

The RECTUS ABDOMINIS of the right fide, (146.) is thrown down like a ftrap over the thigh, fo fully that its tendon by which it is fixed into the Pubis is feen, but not very diftinctly here, becaufe the tendon is fmall, when the Pyramidal Mufcles are found, as in this fubject.

The PYRAMIDAL MUSCLES, (147.) which are as Supplementary Mufcles, are feen fully diffected, with neat, fmall, and flefhy bellies, of a very regular Triangular form; the bafe of the Triangle being the origin of the mufcle from the Pubis; the Apex of the Triangle being its infertion into the LINEA ALBA, and the mark (*) is put upon the place of the Symphifis Pubis.

S 2

PLATE

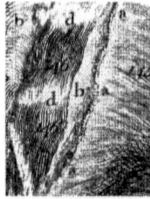

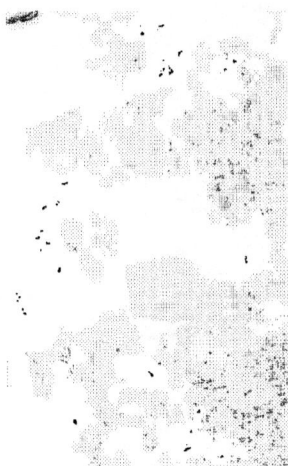

PLATE X.

This Plate explains the Text Book, from Page 323, to Page 328.

THIS drawing explains the Diaphragm in a general way; fhowing how it ftands, " as a Tranfverfe Partition betwixt the Abdomen and the " Thorax;" and how, by its feveral openings, it permits the Veins, Arteries, and great nerves of the Vifcera, to pafs from the one cavity to the other; but ftill it is reprefented here only in a general way; and though its openings are explained, it is rather with the intention of fhowing their places, and their relation to each other, than with any intention of defcribing their particular form; which is more accurately delivered in the next plate.

(1.) Is the upper mufcle of the Diaphragm. This upper and greater mufcle rifes from the inner furface of the Thorax; and befides this origin from the ribs and Sternum, there is alfo another origin, *viz.* from the Ligamentum Arcuatum (*), which ligament is of an arched form, croffing the roots of the QUADRATUS LUMBORUM, (125.) and of the PSOAS MAGNUS (157.); fo that the greater or upper mufcle of the Diaphragm rifes from all the border of the Thorax upon its inner furface, and from this Ligamentum Arcuatum.

3   (2.) The

(2.) The LOWER or POSTERIOR MUSCLE of the Diaphragm rifes from the loins by fmall tendinous heads, which are hidden here by the AORTA (a) paffing over them; but the flefhy part of this lower mufcle is feen with fibres clofely furrounding and embracing the Œfophagus.

(3.) The MIDDLE TENDON is feen, but I do not enter upon the detail, nor pretend to reprefent the croffing of the Tendinous Fibres in this general drawing.

Thus is the Diaphragm, compofed of one great and circular mufcle before, of one fmaller circular mufcle behind, and of the triangular tendon betwixt them; and, both in its flefhy and tendinous parts, it is perforated by feveral veffels, paffing reciprocally between the Thorax and the Abdomen.

Firft, (a) the AORTA, the great artery of the trunk, paffes betwixt the Crura, or legs of the Diaphragm, which like an arch ftrides over it to defend it from preffure.

Secondly, The ŒSOPHAGUS (b), which paffes through the Diaphragm, a little above the Aorta, and a little towards the left fide. Its paffage is by the hole (b) through the lower flefhy belly, and through the moft flefhy part of the Diaphragm, and the mufcular fibres of the Crura Diaphragmatis firft crofs under the hole for the Œfophagus. They furround it, then crofs again above the hole, fo that they form the figure of 8; and the Œfophagus is fo apparently compaffed by thefe furrounding fibres, that fome anatomifts have reckoned this a fort of Sphincter for the upper orifice of the ftomach.

Thirdly, The GREAT VENA CAVA; (c) (both that branch of the Great Vena Cava, which belongs to the Liver, and that alfo, which comes from the lower extremity) goes up to the right fide of the heart, through the right fide of the Diaphragm by the hole (c), where a part of this great vein is feen hanging down with a flaccid and open mouth; and this hole (c), being of a triangular form, paffing in the hard tendon, and being larger than the vein requires, there is no danger of the vein being ftrangulated.

2   (d) Is

(*d*) Is the Left Kidney.

(*e*) Is the Cellular Subftance in the loins, in which the right kidney lies, the kidney of that fide being torn away.

(*f*) Is the Bifurcation of the Aorta a little above the top of the Sacrum, and (*g*) the two Iliac arteries.

(159.) Is the ILIACUS INTERNUS MUSCLE, and (*h*) fhows the manner in which the Iliacus Internus, Pfoas Magnus, and Femoral Artery, come out from under the Femoral Ligament.

The anatomy of the Diaphragm is continued in the next plate.

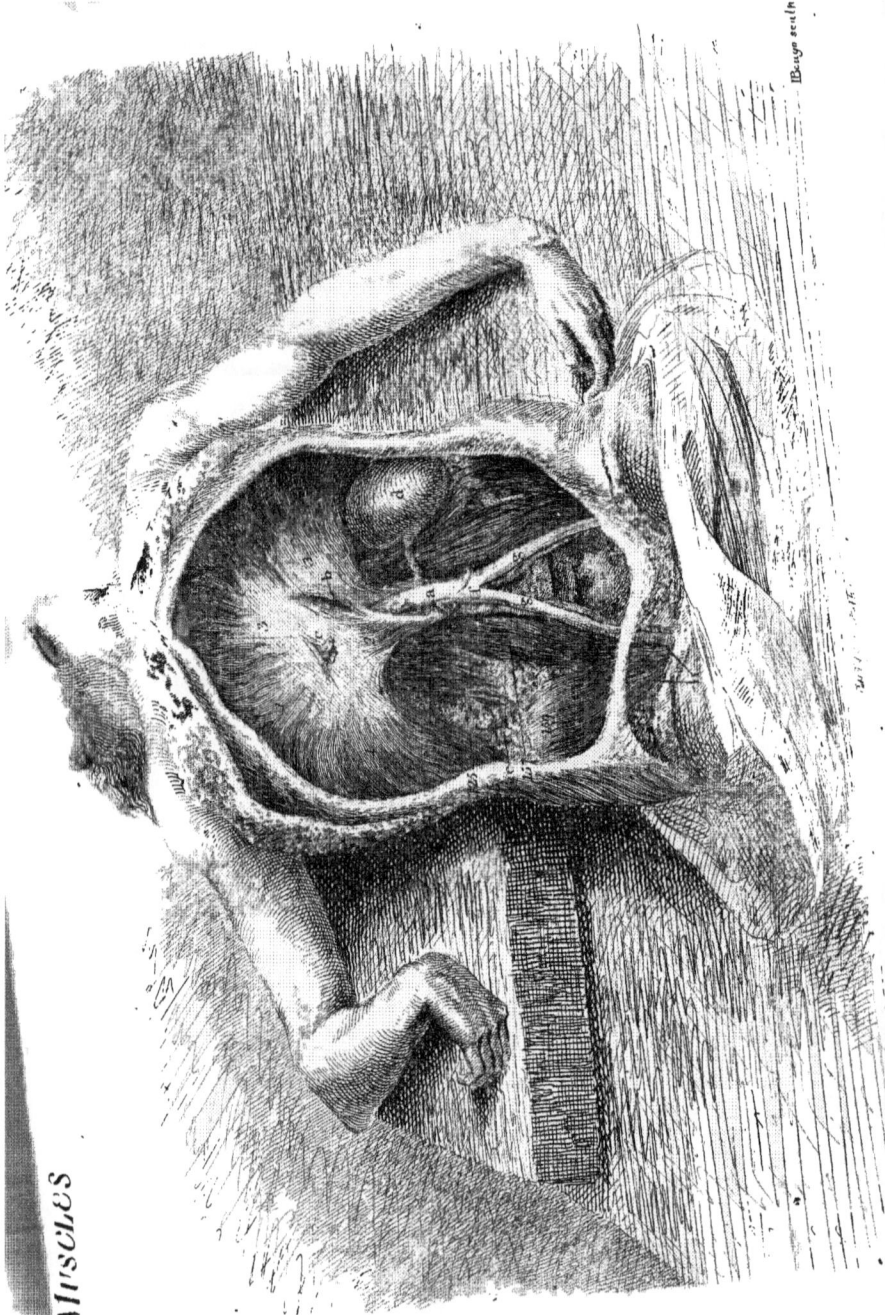

MUSCLES

P L A T E   XI.

This Plate explains the Text Book, from Page 325, to Page 335.

THIS plate confifts of plans of the Diaphragm, and Parts of Generation.

The firft figure is a drawing of the Diaphragm, neatly diffected and taken out of the body; explaining all its origins, and all its holes more correctly than plate x.

The fecond figure is rather a plan than a drawing, and may be very ufeful to the young anatomift, in giving him correct notions of the general form of the Diaphragm, how it ftands flaunting upon the whole; convex towards the cheft, concave towards the belly, and moving (as it may eafily be conceived by this drawing,) fo as to perform refpiration, and all the leffer functions that depend upon it.

And the third figure explains the mufcles which belong to the parts of Generation. This is by no means a plan merely, as might be conceived from the formal fhapes of thefe mufcles, but a true drawing after feveral careful diffections, where, though the parts feem formal, they are really natural, not exaggerated nor caricatured, but delivered fairly and honeftly as they muft always be feen after a right diffection. And they are expofed in fuch a pofture, as by its correfpondence with that

T

for

for Lithotomy will at once convey a leſſon of ſurgery, while it gives correct and true ideas of theſe parts.

FIGURE I.

DRAWING OF THE DIAPHRAGM.

The parts pointed out along with the Diaphragm marked (145.) are parts of the Tranſverſe muſcles of the Abdomen, which, being internal muſcles and riſing from the inner ſurface of the Thorax, have their tongue-like origins (*a a a*), which come from the ribs, mixed confuſedly with (*b b b*), the tongue-like origins of the great muſcle of the Diaphragm, which tongue-like origins (*b b*) come from the ſame ribs; and it was from this connection with the two Tranſverſe Muſcles of the Abdomen, that the Diaphragm was once reckoned a Trigaſtric Muſcle; *Vid.* Book of the Muſcles, page 315.

(1.) The greater, or upper muſcle of the Diaphragm, has theſe five origins; on both ſides (*b b b b*) mark the fleſh which riſes from the ribs, from the inner ſurface of the Thorax, indigitated with the origins of the Tranſverſe Muſcle; (*e e*) mark the two backmoſt portions of the great Anterior Muſcle, and theſe two portions riſe from the two Ligamenta Arcuata, which ſtretch over the origins of the QUADRATUS LUMBORUM and PSOAS Muſcles. And (*f*) marks a fifth portion of the greater muſcle, which riſes from the inner ſurface of the Sternum and Xiphoid Cartilage.

(2.) The leſſer muſcle riſes by four tendinous feet from the fore-part of the Lumbar Vertebræ; and theſe, the CRURA DIAPHRAGMATIS (*g g*), which ſurround the trunk of the Aorta, and their tendinous feet (*h h h*) are very fairly repreſented here, for they are not nicely cut and pared into diſtinct feet, but are repreſented as they are taken up from the face of the Lumbar Vertebræ; that is, not in the ſhape of

3   four

four diſtinct tendons, but adhering to each other in the form of a ſort of denſe tendinous membrane, very white and gliſtening; forming a ſort of ſheath over the fore-parts of the Vertebræ; having flat ſtrings, which are thicker and ſtronger, and more brilliant than the others; but not to be ſeparated (without violence), into the ſhapes of diſtinct feet.

The tendinous feet of the Diaphragm (h h), unite into the Crura at (g g), and the two Crura, growing gradually more fleſhy, form at (i i) the Poſterior Muſcle of the Diaphragm; and it is here, that the fibres of this poſterior or leſſer muſcle croſs and mix, and ſurround the hole for the Œſophagus, with thoſe fibres, which by their croſſing, deſcribe irregularly the figure of eight; and by their compreſſing the Œſophagus form a ſort of Sphincter.

(3.) The CENTRAL TENDON is compoſed of fibres, " which come from the vari" ous Faſciculi of this muſcle, and meet and croſs each other with a confuſed in" ter-lacement which Albinus has been at much pains to trace, but which Haller de" ſcribes much more ſenſibly, as Intricationes variæ, et vix dicendæ; irregular and " confuſed croſſing chiefly at the openings, and eſpecially at the Vena Cava, the " triangular form of which ſeems to be guarded in a moſt particular way." Vid. book, page 327. And the figure (3, 3.) is repeated upon the ſurface of the tendon, to ſhow the various Faſciculæ of the tendinous fibres, which are truely " variæ et " vix dicendæ," and which it were not only difficult, but uſeleſs to deſcribe.

(k) Is the Aorta, where it comes out from the Thorax into the Abdomen; it is here flaccid, and uninjected. Its firſt branches, viz. the Cæliac, and upper Meſenteric Arteries are ſeen going off at this point. It was drawn aſide to ſhow the hole through which it paſſes, and was fixed ſo by a pin.

(l) Is the hole, by which the Œſophagus paſſes, left empty.

(m) Is the hole, by which the Vena Cava paſſes through the tendinous center of the Diaphragm.

T 2

In

FIGURE II.

In this Figure, the Diaphragm is drawn in a new posture; for the trunk (*viz.* the Pelvis and Thorax, with the intermediate Vertebræ of the loins) is set almost upright. And first, the Convexity of the Diaphragm, towards the Thorax (*a*), should be observed. Secondly, the obliquity of the Diaphragm should be observed; its greater muscle rising from all the borders of the Thorax, as at (*b b*), while its Crura and tendinous feet rise near the top of the Pelvis, from the lowest Vertebra of the loins. Thirdly, the true appearance of the tendinous feet is marked, the longest lying in the middle, and the shorter ones being more to the side; so that (*c*), the longest one, lies fair upon the fore-part of the Vertebra of the loins, and rises almost from the lowest Vertebra; while the shortest one (*d*) rises from the Transverse Process of the fourth Vertebra of the loins.

FIGURE III.

The third figure of this plate explains the muscles of the parts **of generation**, the hips and thighs being presented as in the operation of Lithotomy.

For the full explanation of these muscles, the student must turn to the Book of the Muscles, chapter vii. page 329. where he will find that,

(1.) The ERECTOR PENIS (150.) is a delicate and slender muscle about two inches in length, rising from the Tuberosity of the Os Ischium (*a*); lying along the root of the Crus Penis, where it is smallest; inserted into the Crus Penis; being very small, and almost pointed both at its origin, and at its insertion *.

(2.) The

* Haller will not allow this muscle the name of Erector; he says it does not draw the Penis back to the Pubis, but that its office rather is to depress the Penis, and hold it down to the proper angle,

for

(2.) The TRANSVERSALIS PERINÆI, (151.) rifes along with the Erector; from the Tuber Ifchii (a), it croffes the deep hollow which is betwixt the Ifchium and the Anus; and is fixed into the backmoft point of the bulb of the Urethra.

(3.) The ACCELERATOR URINÆ, (152.) is a double mufcle; or a pair of mufcles one lying upon each fide of the bulb of the Urethra, fo that the whole fairly furrounds the bulb. And indeed this tumor of the bulb feems chiefly formed to favour the action of the Accelerator Mufcle; and the two flender and horn-like tendons of the Accelerator are feen plainly turning off from the cavernous body of the Urethra (b) to go out upon the cavernous body of the Crus Penis (c), by which hold it plays more powerfully upon the bulb. We feel the actions of this mufcle very plainly in the throwing out of the laft drops of urine, as well as in the ejaculation of the Semen; and its great power of throwing the Semen to a diftance has been afcertained by experiments, fuch as fhould not be repeated. nor mentioned, indeed, except in that language in which they were told. " Conftat enim per experimenta, ob turpitudinem " non repetenda, multo longius femen de fano et dudum cafto homine profelire " quam abeft uterus." The SPHINCTER ANI (153.), is feen furrounding the opening of the Anus.

Wounds of thefe mufcles are attended with no degree of danger, nor followed by any kind of incapacity, but yet it is very manifeft, that fince the incifions for Lithotomy fhould be made in one regular and uniform line, thefe mufcles will be cut by every dextrous operator in one certain way; and the naming them wrong muft be a mark either of ignorance of thefe parts, or at the leaft, of a bad irregular operation. Now, as the aim of the Lithotomift is to get into the bladder by that great hollow which lies betwixt the Tuberofity of the Os Ifchium (a), and the Anus (d); the incifion muft pafs exactly in the middle betwixt the Tuber and the Anus.

for entering the Vagina. What a pity it is that the illuftrious author had not afcertained this curious angle! for we fhould naturally conceive, at leaft from what we fee after our injections, that the Penis when in full erection, ftood up to the Pubis as clofe as it could lie.

Anus. The Tranfverfalis Perinœi muft be fairly cut acrofs; the Accelerator will be fpared; the Erector cannot be cut; and the operator who cuts the Accelerator, keeps his knife too near the Anus, and wounds the bulb. The operator who fpeaks of cutting the Erector, either muft be very ignorant of this fame Erector, or muft intend to cut upon the Tuberofity of the Ifchium, hoping perhaps to cut through the bone: But what fhall we think of a furgeon, who fpeaks about things of this kind fo loofely, as to talk of cutting both the Erector and the Accelerator Mufcle; that is of cutting both that mufcle which lies on the outfide of the common incifion, and alfo that one which lies on the infide of the common incifion? After reading this in any author, one might be inclined to turn backwards a page or two, to fee whether he made an incifion like that of Celfus; viz. in the fhape of a half-moon.

PLATE

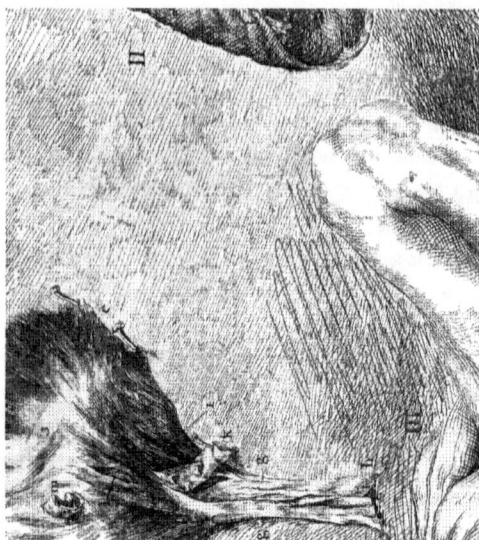

PLATE XII.

This Plate and the next explain the Text Book, from Page 336, to Page 384.

OF THE LOWER EXTREMITY.

IN this plate are explained the chief mufcles of the Thigh, Leg, and Foot.
The limb is hung by a rope, the foot fwinging in the air, the ball of
the great toe touching the ground. The leg is prefented twice. In a fore
view fhewing the great fafcia of the thigh diffected back, and the mufcles naked, Fig. i.   And again, in a back view, Fig. ii. fhewing the
cavity of the Pelvis; the hollow betwixt the Ham-ftring mufcles, and
the bellies of the Gaftrocnæmii with the great Achilles Tendon.
The explanations cannot be orderly, and therefore they fhould be
fhort.

In FIGURE I. (*a*) marks the Spine of the Ilium ; (*b*) the creft of the Pubis ; (*c*) the ligament of Paupart which runs betwixt thefe two points ; (*d*) the Femoral artery paffing under the ligament.   The mufcles which appear on the fore-part of the thigh
are thefe.

The RECTUS (171.) lying in the middle of the thigh, having a white and tendinous
part in the center, and the flefhy fibres going in towards it.

                                                                        The

The Vastus Externus (173.) making all the flesh on the the outside of the thigh.

The Vastus Internus (174.) making that cushion of flesh, which is so prominent upon the inner side of the knee joint, and which makes so particular a mark in the drawings of the thigh : and all these three muscles, viz. the Rectus, Vastus Externus, and Vastus Internus, are inserted together into the Patella, which is marked (e).

Then the Sartorius 175.) is seen rising from the highest point of the Os Ilium ; crossing the thigh, long and slender like a strap, and bending down the Vastus Internus Muscle.

The head of the Gracilis (176.) where it rises from the Pubis is here seen ;—next to that is seen the first head of the Triceps (161.) ; and next to that the Pectinalis (160.) with the artery of the thigh lying flat upon its belly.

These are the chief muscles on the fore part of the thigh ; they are naturally covered with the Fascia, or broad tendinous expansion, marked (f), and the Fascialis Muscle, which, from its making this vagina tense, is named Tensor Vaginæ Femoris ; is marked with its appropriated number (156.), and is drawn out along with the fascia, and is seen rising from the same point of the Os Ilium, from which the Sartorius rises.

In the Leg, (g) marks the Tibia ; and the muscles are,

The Gastrocnæmius, (181.)

The Tibialis Anticus (187.), which comes from the fore part of the Tibia, crosses the ancle obliquely, goes over the side of the foot to be implanted into the root of the great toe ; and this is the tendon which makes that sharp angle on the fore-part of the ancle where the buckle lies.

The Extensor Pollicis (196.) lies next to the Tibialis, and its tendon passes like that of the Tibialis Anticus under the Annular Ligament of the ancle, which is marked (b) ; and next to the Extensor Pollicis lies the Extensor Longus Digitorum Pedis (193.) which lies deeper still, and more towards the outside of the leg. Its tendons are seen going out to each of the toes, and these tendons are accompanied with the

3   tendons

tendons of the little mufcle the EXTENSOR BREVIS DIGITORUM PEDIS (195.),
   which is feen lying under the tendons of the long mufcle.

Behind the Extenfor Digitorum, and hiding it in part, is the PERONEUS LONGUS Mufcle
   (184.), which belongs to the brawn of the Leg, and the tendon of which paffes down
   behind the outer ancle.

In the foot, Fig. II. lying under this one, is explained the Plantar Aponeurofis, or that
   fafcia which belongs to the fole of the foot; and which is defcribed in the Book of
   Mufcles, page 382. It is feen here to confift of three general divifions, the middle one
   (i), the lateral one (k) on the outfide, which covers the Flexor, and the Abdu&or
   Minimi Digiti; and the lateral one (l) on the infide, which covers the Flexor and
   the Abdu&or Pollicis.

The general Fafcia where it covers the thigh is marked (f), but it is merely a continuation of the fame fafcia that covers the leg; and where it covers the leg it is
   marked (*); and it is ftill the fame fafcia which being continued over the fore-part
   of the foot, is there ftrengthened by its adhefion to the outer and inner ancles, by
   which, taking a new form it becomes the Annular Ligament, fo that the Annular
   Ligament is merely a ftrengthening of the common fafcia.

FIGURE III.

THIS view fhows chiefly the mufcles upon the back part of the thigh and leg. The
   Vertical Se&ion of the Os Sacrum is marked (m); the hollow of the Pelvis is
   marked (n); the Vertical Se&ion of the Os Pubis is marked (o); and the letter
   (p) is put down upon the Tuberofity of the Os Ifchium, which could not be clearly marked. And the mufcles are,

The PSOAS MAGNUS (157.); croffing the brim of the Pelvis, to go down into the thigh.

The GRACILIS (176.), which is feen coming from the arch of the Pubis, and going down
   to be inferted by a delicate and flender tendon, into the head of the Tibia.

U   The

The firſt and ſecond heads of the TRICEPS, (161.) are ſeen from behind.

The SEMI-MEMBRANOSUS (178.) is next ſeen; but the whole of it is not ſeen; nothing is bare here but the middle and lower parts of the muſcle; but there is enough of it to ſhow that it is not as its name imports, a muſcle having a membranous appearance, it has on the contrary a very thick fleſhy belly.

The SEMI-TENDINOSUS (177.) is next to it, and the reaſon of its being named Semi-tendi-noſus is ſeen in the length of its tendon (q). The Semi-membranoſus and the Semi-tendinoſus form together the inner ham-ſtring. The outer ham-ſtring is formed by the Tendon of the Biceps Cruris Muſcle; and the belly of the Biceps (180.) is ſeen held out by three ſticks, ſo as to ſhow the deep hollow betwixt the ham-ſtrings, in which is ſeen hanging the great SACRO-SCIATIC NERVE (r); where it is going down the back of the thigh, to paſs down under the heads of the Gaſtrocnemii Muſcles.

The GREAT GLUTÆUS MUSCLE (163.) is ſeen upon the hip diſſected, ſo as to ſhow the order of its fibres, and hanging like the reſt of the leg all looſe and flaccid.

The VASTUS INTERNUS (174.) is alſo ſeen making a fleſhy belly juſt over the knee-joint.

The two bellies of the GASTROCNEMIUS MUSCLE (181.) are ſeen riſing each from its own Condyle of the thigh bone at (s s), and meeting together to be joined into the great Achillis tendon (t); which grows gradually ſmaller as it goes downwards to be im-planted into the heel at (u), where ſtill it is very thick and ſtrong.

The great belly and tendon of the FLEXOR POLLICIS (188.) is alſo ſeen paſſing behind the inner ancle.

A part of the belly of the SOLÆUS (182.) is ſeen lying under the belly of the Gaſtro-cnemius.

The foot in this drawing, is left covered with ſkin, and puffed, and ill ſhaped, as it naturally is, while under diſſection.

PLATE

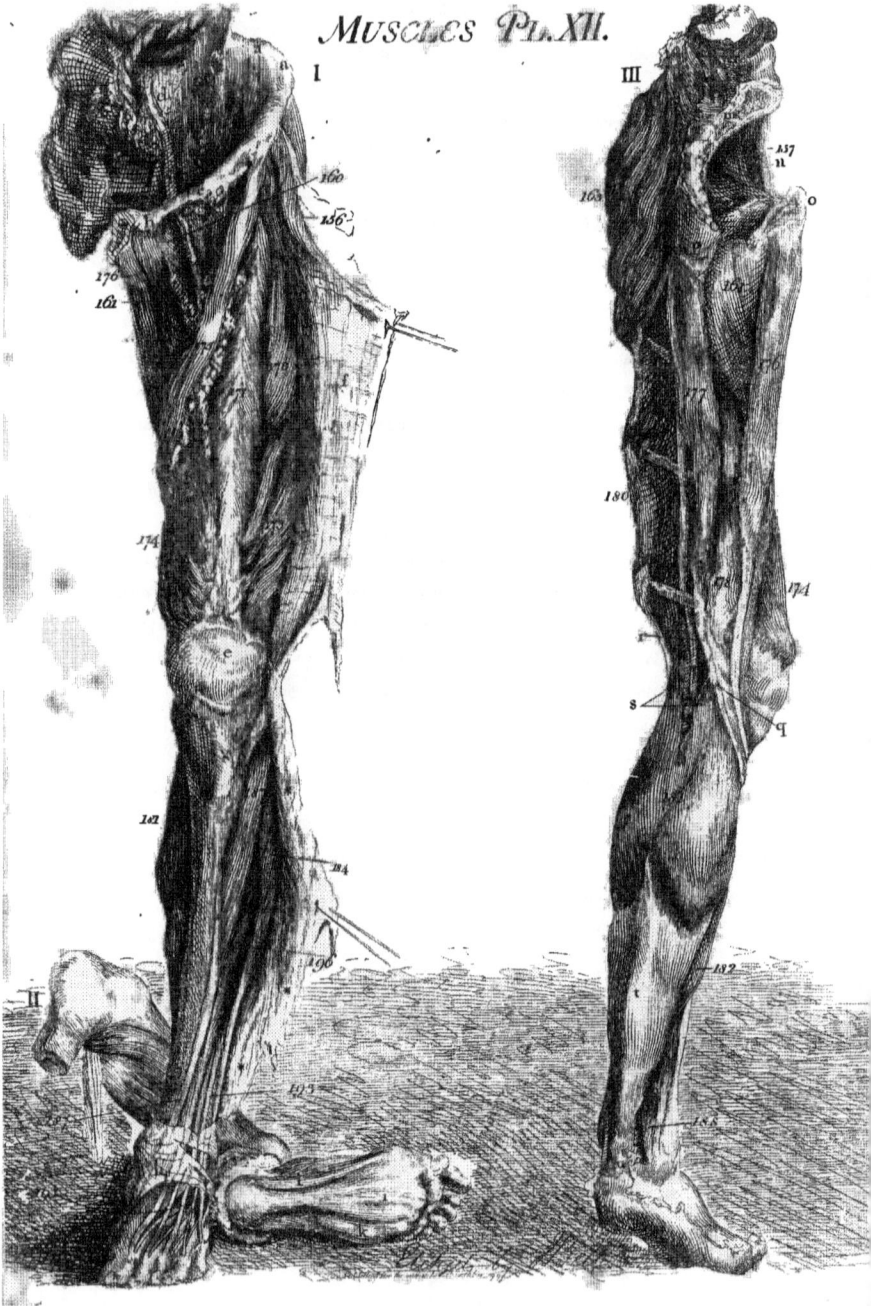

MUSCLES Pl.XII.

PLATE XIII.

This Plate explains the Text Book, from Page 336, to Page 384.

SHOWS the deeper mufcles of the THIGH, LEG, and FOOT, alfo in two drawings; one reprefenting the fore, and the other the back-parts of the leg. This is a fuller diffection than the laft, fo that it differs greatly in general appearance from the laft drawing, but ftill the general pofition is exactly the fame.

In FIGURE I. are feen,

The GLUTÆUS MAXIMUS (163.) now diffected, and cut away from its origin in the haunch bone, left at its infertion into the thigh bone. It is hung out by a ftring, and the fhape, which it falls into, fnows that it is one of the heavieft and flefhieft mufcles in the body; a part of the Glutæus Medius (164.) is feen under it.

The RECTUS FEMORIS (171.) is now cut away, and nothing of it is left here, but its origin from the Spinous Procefs marked (a); and its infertion into the Patella, which is marked (b) is thrown down and left hanging. By the throwing down of the RECTUS FEMORIS, the great mafs of the CRURÆUS (172.) which lies under it is expofed, and it is feen that the Cruræus confifts partly of tendon, partly of flefh, extends all along the thigh, rifes from the thigh bone, lies immediately under the Rectus, and is inferted along with it into the Patella; and here the VASTUS EXTER-

U 2   NUS

NUS (173.) is feen in its place. The VASTUS INTERNUS (174.) is cut and thrown down, and left hanging over the knee like the Rectus.

The SARTORIUS (175.) is also cut away from the Ilium, and left hanging down along the leg.

The FASCIALIS (156.) is feen here also with a rag of its fascia connected with it.

The PSOAS MAGNUS (157.) which comes from the fides of the Lumbar Vertebræ, and the ILIACUS INTERNUS (159.) which comes from the infide of the haunch bone, are feen turning over the fore-part of the Pelvis together to go down through among the flesh of the thigh, to the leffer or inner Trochanter of the thigh bone.

The PECTINALIS (160.) is feen rifing from the Pubis, and ftretching flat and direct towards the thigh bone.

The TRICEPS LONGUS marked (1.), as it is the firft head of the Triceps Femoris, (161.) is feen here thick, and flefhy. This covers the other two heads of the Triceps, viz. the Triceps Brevis, and Triceps Magnus; the edge of the TRICEPS MAGNUS, or third head of the Triceps, is feen here, (3.); but the TRICEPS BREVIS or fecond head of the Triceps is here entirely covered by the Pectinalis and Triceps Longus, and is feen only in the fecond drawing, where it is marked (2.)

The mufcles on the back-parts of the hip and thigh, are explained in figures ii. and iii. iv.

In FIGURE II. we have the GLUTÆUS MAXIMUS (163.) hung out by a ftring as in the other drawing. The PSOAS MAGNUS (157.) croffing the brim of the Pelvis as in the former drawings; the Triceps Longus marked (1.) defcending from the Pubis, to the middle of the thigh bone; behind that is feen the Triceps Brevis, vel fecundus, (2.) the fecond head of the Triceps, which is held as a part of the fame mufcle, though it lies behind the firft, and is of a different layer; and behind that ftill lies the TRICEPS Magnus (3.), which has alfo very little connection with the other heads, but it is called the third head of the Triceps; and there is feen the Femoral Artery marked (c) paffing through the Triceps Magnus from the fore to the back part of the thigh; the artery is marked (c), and the tendon of the Triceps Magnus, where it is implanted

ed into the inner Condyle of the thigh bone, is marked (*d*); fo that the artery paffes through the Triceps from the fore to the back part of the thigh, only a little above the knee.

The root of the Semi-membranofus (178.) is feen at (*e*), where it rifes by a thick and flefhy head from the Tuberofity of the Os Ifchium; the lower end of it where it is attached to the head of the Tibia is cut, and hangs down at (*f*).

The oppofite Ham-ftring Mufcle the Biceps (180.) is feen; its bellies are marked with the proper number of the mufcle. Its longer head is feen rifing in common with the Semi-membranofus from the Tuberofity of the Os Ifchium at (*g*); the longer head is marked (*g*), but the fhorter head of the Biceps which rifes from the back of the thigh bone, is marked (*b*); the place where the long and the fhort heads of the Biceps Femoris unite and mix their fibres is marked (*i*); and the tendon of the Biceps which forms the outer ham-ftring is marked (*k*).

All the ham, or the back part of the knee-joint, is now expofed by the throwing down of the conjoined mufcles, the GASTROCNEMIUS EXTERNUS (181.) and the SOLÆUS, (182.) which are left only at their infertion by the great Achillis Tendon (*l*), which is fixed into the heel bone; and the Gaftrocnemius and Solæus being thus thrown down, the two curious mufcles which lie in the ham are expofed, *viz.* the PLANTARIS (183.) which rifes from the outer Condyle of the Os Femoris, has a very fmall delicate flefhy belly, like that of the PALMARIS LONGUS. It has alfo a fmall round tendon like it, the fmalleft and longeft in the body, not groffer than a fiddle-ftring; which going down along the inner furface of the Gaftrocnæmius, and making an impreffion upon the inner furface of the great Achillis Tendon, accompanies it to the heel, where it is implanted along with it.

The other fmall mufcle is the proper mufcle of the ham, which is thence named MUS-CULUS POPLITÆUS (179.) It is a beautiful triangular mufcle, which lies exactly upon the back part of the joint as a fort of guard to the Capfule, and like a check band for fupporting the knee. It comes from the outer Condyle along with the

little

little belly of the Plantaris, croſſes the joint with oblique fibres; comes from the Condyle of the thigh bone; is inſerted into the back of the Tibia, and ſo bends the knee.

In the legs of both drawings, the following deep ſeated muſcles are ſeen. In the firſt leg, the deep muſcles of the toes which lie under the Tibialis Anticus, and they are all extenſors of the toes. In the ſecond leg the deep muſcles which lie under the Gaſtrocnemius and Solæus; and they are all flexors of the toes.

In Figure I. is ſeen (m), the place upon the fore-part of the Tibia, from which the fleſhy belly of the Tibialis Anticus is cut away, ſo that the next muſcle the Extensor Pollicis (196.) is ſeen, which is a long, penniform, and very ſtrong muſcle; and its long tendon is ſeen going to the great toe.

Behind that again, lies the Extensor Longus Digitorum Pedis (193.), which has its fleſhy belly lying behind the Extenſor Pollicis; and its four tendons are raiſed over one leg of the compaſſes, ſo as to expoſe the ſhort flexor which lies beneath, upon that part of the foot where the buckle reſts; and which is ſeen beginning by a ſmall head (n), from the heel bone. Behind the Extenſor Digitorum lies a third muſcle, which is like a ſlip of the Extenſor, but its tendon does not run into the toes. It is fixed into the ſide of the foot at the root of the little toe, it is therefore a bender of the foot, and from its riſing from the Fibula, is named Peroneus Tertius (194.)

And Laſtly, in this figure, a part of the Peroneus Longus (184.) is ſeen, a muſcle which rightly belongs to the other ſide of the leg, and the tendon of which paſſes behind the outer ancle, to go down into the ſole of the foot.

In Figure II. are ſeen, in like manner, all the long flexors of the toes and foot.

Firſt the Tibialis Posticus (186.) begins with a ſtrong fleſhy belly upon the back part of the Tibia; is penniform like moſt of theſe long muſcles of the leg; and ſends a long tendon down behind the inner ancle, which runs in a particular ring of the Ligaments that are behind the ancle; and, getting into the ſole of the foot, is fixed by many ſpreading roots into the ſeveral bones of the Tarſus.

The

The FLEXOR LONGUS DIGITORUM PEDIS (189.) lies immediately behind this; is like it in all points; sends its long slender tendon down also behind the ancle in its own peculiar ring, but, passing the bones of the Tarsus, it divides into four tendons, which go to each of the lesser toes.

The FLEXOR LONGUS POLLICIS PEDIS (188.) is the appropriated muscle of the great toe. It has a large fleshy belly, a very strong big tendon, and runs by the inner ancle in its own peculiar ring. Now it is to be noticed, that this Flexor Pollicis, though the flexor only of one single toe, is much bigger than the common flexor of all the toes. It is even bigger than both these, or the Tibialis Posticus, which is the great muscle of the foot. The meaning of which is very plain; viz. that these muscles of the toes are to be considered not so much as mere benders of the toes; for when we observe how little the toes move, and how much walking consists in rising upon the ball of the great toe, we shall regard these muscles rather as benders of the whole foot. It is by the power of these muscles, that we beat the ground in each step in walking, for in walking each push in carrying the body is made by the pressing of the ball of the great toe against the ground; and these muscles all press down the ball of the great toe. In making the step, these flexor muscles of the toe, and foot, are chiefly assisted by a muscle belonging to the other side of the leg, I mean the PE- RONEUS LONGUS (184.), which rises not like these, from the back of the Tibia, to pass behind the inner ancle, but from the whole length of the Fibula, whence its name of Peroneus, and passes down in a ring behind the outer ancle; and this strong tendon which makes the sharpness behind the outer ancle, and gives shape to the leg, is here drawn out with a string just where it is descending into its sheath or ring.

Thus all the muscles which bend the foot, and so raise the body at each step, are distinctly seen in this dissection; viz. The GASTROCNEMIUS (181.) the SOLÆUS (182.) and the PLANTARIS (183.); the TIBIALIS POSTICUS (186.) FLEXOR DIGITORUM (189.) FLEXOR POLLICIS (188.) and PERONEUS LONGUS. (184.) There is but one more, the

X   Peroneus

Peroneus Brevis, which is fo exactly like the Peroneus Longus, that its not being feen in this view, is hardly an imperfection, the demonstration being fufficiently full.

The foot is diffected in Figure iii. where is feen firft the fhort Flexor, the FLEXOR BREVIS DIGITORUM PEDIS (191.), cut up from the heel bone where it has its origin; its flefhy belly is thrown out; its fhort neat tendons are going to each of the toes; its tendons are perforated like thofe of the hand, for the tranfmiffion of the tendons of the long Flexor. The tendons of the long Flexor are marked (o); they are feen going forwards to thread the loops, made by the fhort tendons; and there is feen connected with the long Flexor that fhort fupplementary mufcle which comes from the heel bone, and which being irregular in its form, is called the MASSA CARNEA JACOBI SILVII (190.). The Lumbricales are too delicate to be feen in a fmall drawing like this, but they are eafily found in diffection, for they are like a continuation of the Maffa Carnea lying in the forks of the tendons.

The tendon of the long Flexor of the great toe is feen here (p), efcaping from under the inner ancle, and appearing upon the fole of the foot; and it is feen to be connected here (by a fmall flip of tendon) with the long Flexor of all the toes. This tendon of the long Flexor of the great toe is feen to pafs betwixt the two heads of the fhort flexor, which is marked with its proper number (191.) The Abductor of the little toe is alfo feen.

There remain to be explained, certain mufcles which immediately furround the hip joint; and which are defcribed in the book from page 347, to 352.

The TROCHANTERS are fo named, becaufe they are placed fo that moft of the mufcles which are implanted into them, at the fame time that they bend the thigh, turn it alfo.

Thefe mufcles are explained by figure iv. The Pelvis is hung up by a rope, put round the Lumbar Vertebræ; and the points of bone to be obferved as explaining the pofture are, (q) the line of the Os Sacrum, and Os Coccygis; (r) the tuberofity

x   of

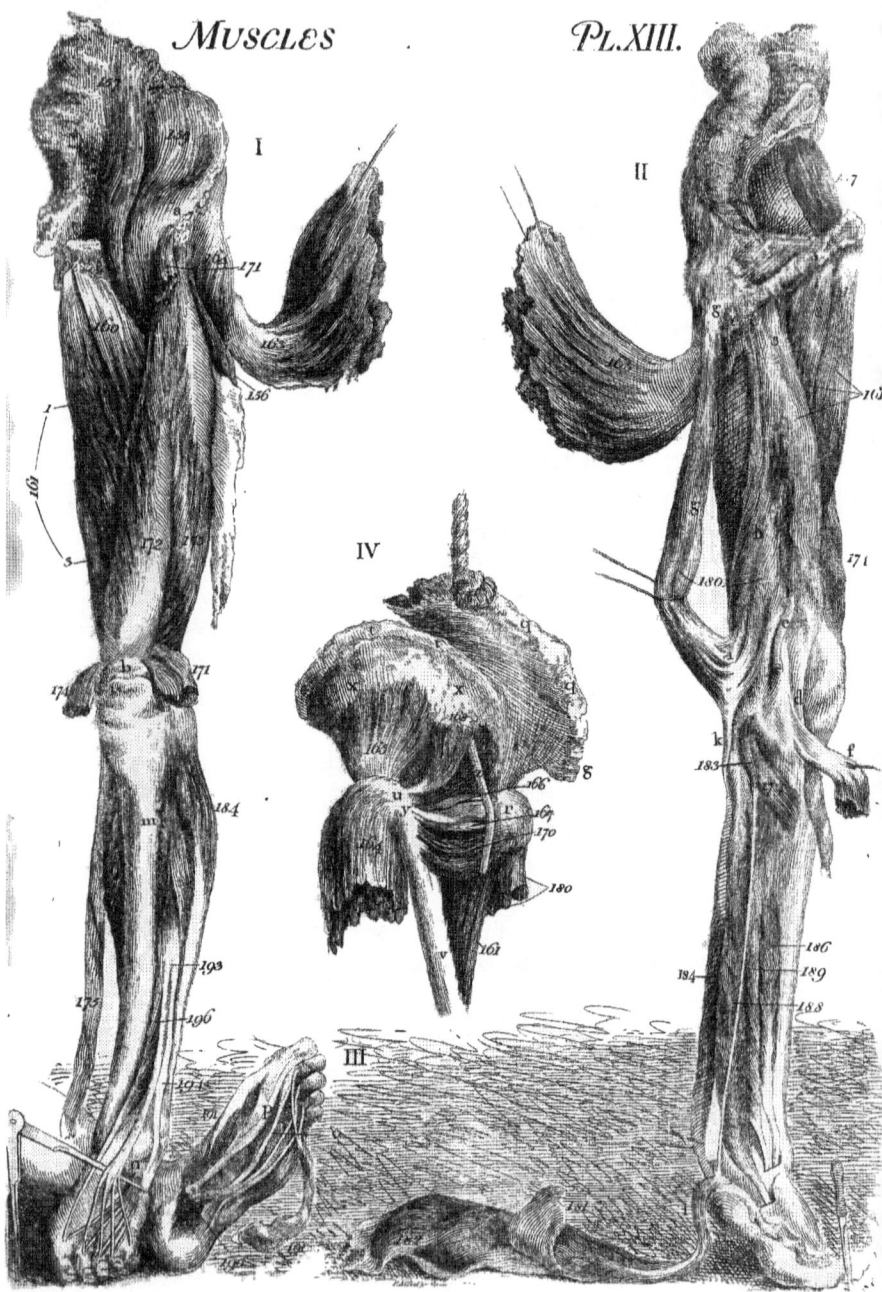

MUSCLES   PL.XIII.

of the Os Ifchium; (*s*) the Sacro-Sciatic Ligament paffing from the Sacrum, to the
Ifchium; (*t*) the Spine of the Ilium; (*u*) the great Trochanter of the Thigh
Bone; and (*v*) the fhaft of the fame bone.

And the mufcles that are feen are,

FIRST, the GLUTÆUS MEDIUS (164.) cut away from its origin, which is from the
Os Ilium at (*x*); the great Glutæus, which rifes from the Sacrum and Ilium,
from (*g*) to (*t*) being cut entirely away. The middle Glutæus (164.) is feen to be
implanted into the very Apex of the Trochanter; the GLUTÆUS MINIMUS (165.)
which lies under it, rifes again from that part of the Os Ilium that forms the
focket for the Thigh Bone; and is of courfe the deepeft, and the fmalleft of thefe
mufcles.

Behind the GLUTÆUS MINIMUS is feen the PYRIFORMIS (168.); and the reafon of its
name, taken from its Pyramidal form, is well explained; and its broad thin belly is
feen coming from the hollow of the Sacrum within the Cavity of the Pelvis; and
its fmall flat tendon is feen inferted into the root of the Trochanter Major.

The QUADRATUS FEMORIS, (170.) a fhort and fquare mufcle is feen coming from the
tuberofity of the Os Ifchium, and implanted into the greater Trochanter.

The mufcles, named Marfupiales, are feen going into the Trochanter at the point
marked (*y*); and I do not put their right numbers (166.) (167.) upon them,
left it fhould confound fo fmall a drawing. Befides, it will be eafily enough underftood, that the white tendon, marked (*y*), is the tendon of the Obturator Internus, which comes from within the Pelvis, turning over the tuberofity of the Os
Ifchium; and the little flefhy flips above and below this white tendon, and inclof-
ing it upon either fide, are the GEMINI MUSCLES (166.) (167.), one above, another
below the Obturator Internus, and all the three inferted together into the root of
the Trochanter at the point (*y*). A part of the TRICEPS FEMORIS is marked (161.);
the heads of the Biceps, and of the Semi-tendinofus, and Semi-membranofus

X

where

where they all three rife together from the tuberofity of the Os Ifchium, have
the mark of the Biceps only, which is (180.)

The SACRO-SCIATIC NERVE, where it comes out from the cavity of the Pelvis, along
with the Pyriform Mufcle, is marked (∗).

THE

THIRD BOOK,

OF THE

JOINTS.

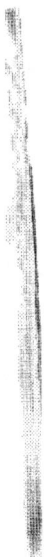

B O O K T H I R D.

OF THE

J O I N T S.

———————— • ————————

IF this book feem fhort, it is becaufe I have omitted many joints, which
it is decent and proper for the profeffed anatomift to be acquainted with,
but which it were very fuperfluous to trouble the ftudent about, for the
fubject is hardly even curious, and certainly not ufeful. Therefore
I have made a fuller defcription of the fhoulder, knee, and hip; and
have refrained from giving any drawings of the joints of the head, of
the Vertebræ, or of the ribs; for thefe joints are not eafily underftood, are hardly worth remembering, and are very foon forgotten.
It was natural for me to be afraid left the hiftory and drawings of
thefe joints might fwell the book, making it more expenfive, and lefs
ufeful.

PLATE

P L A T E   I.

This Plate explains the Text Book, from Page 427, to Page 439.

EXPLAINS the Shoulder Joint, Elbow, and Wrist.

FIGURE   I.

IS the shoulder joint which was set up for this drawing, the whole piece of anatomy resting upon the lower angle of the Scapula, and upon the cut end of the Os Humeri. The marked points by which the muscles and the joint are explained, are these chiefly : (*a*) The Clavicle ; the letter (*a*) is placed on the middle of the bone, where it projects in the collar or root of the neck ; (*b*) is the end next the Sternum with some ragged flesh hanging from it ; (*c*) is the flat end by which it touches the point of the Acromion Process ; (*d*) marks the Acromion Process where the Clavicle is joined to it ; and (*e*) is the point or apex of the Coracoid Process. (*f*) Marks that line of the Scapula which is called its base, and it, like the Clavicle, has the remains of its ragged muscle hanging down from it. And lastly, (*g*) is the Os Humeri.

The muscles which are seen here are,

The SUBSCAPULARIS (77.) covering the whole of the Lower Surface of the Scapula, and better explained than in the smaller drawings for the muscles of the arm. A small part of the SUPRA-SPINATUS (73.) is also seen.

The

The Biceps (78.) is marked in the bellies with its proper number, and its two heads
are also marked; the shorter head (*h*) rising from the Coracoid Process; and the
longer head (*i*), coming down from within the cavity of the joint.

The Coraco-Brachialis (72.), is seen hanging down loose and flaccid, from the Coracoid Process, and passing obliquely under the two heads of the Biceps; to be fixed
into the arm bone.

The DELTOIDES (71.) is cut away from the Scapula and turned backwards, and it
hangs over the arm bone very thick and massy. And this white and shining appearance upon the inner surface of the Deltoides is from the Cellular Substance
which lies under it being condensed into somewhat of the form of a fascia. And
it is from this fascia, that one of the great Bursæ Mucosæ belonging to this joint
rises. The flesh of the Deltoid is seen at (*b*), and the fascia, covering the face of
the muscle, is marked with the number (71.) And lastly, the LATISSIMUS DORSI
(70.) is seen cut off about six inches from its insertion into the shoulder bone, and
left hanging there. (*kk*) Wherever they are found, denote the fat which lies in the
interstices of the muscles, and which should not be too curiously picked away in
any part of a dissection, unless it be necessary for making some important part
very clean and distinct.

The parts more immediately belonging to the joint are these.

1. The Acromion Process (*d*) overhangs the joint from above, and prevents luxations
upwards.

2. The Coracoid Process (*e*) stands up on the inside of the arm, to strengthen the
joint in that direction also.

3. The LIGAMENTUM PROPRIUM TRIANGULARE SCAPULÆ (*m*) crosses from the Acromion to the Coracoid Process, makes a sort of bridge betwixt them, and keeps
all firm in that direction.

4. Another ligament is seen here, the LIGAMENTUM COMMUNE TRAPEZOIDES (*n*),
which does not rightly belong to this joint, being but a ligament of the Clavicle;

so

so that there are the following parts attached to the Coracoid Procefs (*e*), *viz.* the Coraco-brachialis (72.), and the fhort head of the biceps (*b*), going down from it, the Ligamentum Triangulare Proprium (*m*) going to the Acromion, and the Ligamentum Commune (*n*) going to the Clavicle.

The Capfule or bag of the joint which is exceedingly thin, and lax, is marked (*o o*); and it is cut open to fhow the head of the bone, as it lies in its focket. This fhows alfo the long tendon (*i*), of the ~~Coraco-brachialis~~ *Biceps* as it comes through the focket, lying upon the round head of the fhoulder bone. And laftly, the flat tendon of the Subfcapularis is feen fpreading over the Capfular Ligament at (*p*), by which it will be eafily conceived, how the other mufcles fpread over the Capfule to ftrengthen it; for here it is feen, that the cut edge of the Capfule, and the cut edge of the tendon of the Subfcapularis is one and the fame part; that is, the flat tendon and the Capfule are fo incorporated, that the one cannot be cut nor torn without the other. And thus it may be underftood, how the chief fecurity and ftrength of the fhoulder joint is from the mufcles furrounding its Capfule fo clofely, and being implanted directly into the head of the bone.

FIGURE II.

Is intended chiefly for fhowing the fhallownefs of the Glenoid Cavity, when compared with the head of the bone, and it alfo explains very well the way in which the long tendon of the biceps rifes from the margin of the Glenoid Cavity.

The SCAPULA (A) is naked, but with the remains of ragged flefh hanging about it; where (*c*) marks the Spine of the Scapula rifing towards (*d*), which is the point of the Acromion Procefs; (*e*) marks the apex of the Coracoid Procefs fcarcely feen; (*m*) is the Ligamentum Proprium Triangulare lying rather in fhadow; the Capfule is here alfo marked (*o o*); it is cut up and thrown quite back in a fquare

3   form

form from the manner in which it is cut; the edges of the cut Capfule are ftill feen furrounding the fhoulder bone, as well as the Glenoid Cavity; and this throwing back of the Capfule fhows the fhallownefs of the Glenoid Cavity (*p*), and the roundnefs and largenefs of the head of the fhoulder bone; and within the Capfule is feen the long head (*i*) of the biceps, rifing from the margin of the focket, at its upper part. (*k*) Marks the remains of the tendon of the Supra-fpinatus Mufcle, where it lies upon the Capfule and adheres to it; and it is this tendon which gives the Capfule an appearance of thicknefs, and makes it turn fo rigidly backwards at this particular point (*k*).

F I G U R E   III.

MAY be compared with figure i. to obferve how entirely the joint is furrounded with its great mufcles : For here is the Infra-fpinatus covering the Capfule, juft as the Subfcapularis does in figure i. But the chief ufe of this figure is to give a true notion of one of the greateft Burfæ Mucofæ that belong to the fhoulder joint.

The Parts marked in this drawing are,

The bafis of the Scapula (*a*); the beginning of the Spine of the Scapula (*b*); the Acromion Procefs (*c*); the Clavicle (*d*); the ligament which ties the outer end of the clavicle firmly to the point of the Acromion Procefs (*e*); the point or apex of the Coracoid Procefs (*f*); the fhaft of the fhoulder bone (*g*). But the head of the fhoulder bone is concealed by the mufcles, and other foft parts.

Then, of the foft parts there are feen chiefly thefe, The great belly of the INFRA-SPINA-TUS Mufcle (74.), where it lies upon the Scapula black and fhining; (for every mufcle when' diffected clean, has a metally-like furface);—the belly of the TERES MINOR (75.), the tendon of which twifts to be implanted thus into the fhoulder bone at (*k*).

The fhort head of the biceps (*b*) is feen rifing from the point of the Coracoid Procefs

Y   (*f*);

(*f*) ; while its longer head (*i*) is seen coming out round and small from the cavity of the joint: The flesh of the CORACO-BRACHIALIS (72.) is seen black, and lying in shadow behind the two heads of the biceps. The two heads of the biceps are not joined to each other till they pass the middle of the arm, *i. e.* below the point where (78.) the number of the biceps is placed.

Lastly, The chief point in this drawing is the Bursa Mucosa marked (*m*) ; which lies on the outside of the Capsular Ligament of the joint ; it is very large, and is surrounded by many smaller ones. This is sufficient to explain the appearance of a Bursa Mucosa ; the use of this great one, lying betwixt the Capsule of the joint and the Acromion Process is easily conceived, and the nature of the smaller ones lying under the point of the Coracoid Process, and under each of the tendons, as of the Teres Major, Latissimus Dorsi, &c. need hardly be explained *.

FIGURE IV.

Explains the Elbow-joint ; and also shows the Wrist, but imperfectly.

The three bones which form the Elbow-joint are, the Humerus (*a*) ; the Radius (*b*) ; and the Ulna (*c*). They are all connected with each other by the general Capsule or bag of the joint (*d*), which is derived from the Periosteum, coming off from the shoulder bone above those hollows which receive the Olecranon and Coronoid Processes ; which is in itself thin, and delicate, but is crossed by lateral and Transverse Ligaments, so that it does not appear like a distinct bag ; and therefore the chief demonstration is of the bands, which go across the Capsular Ligament to strengthen it in various directions.

1. The CORONARY LIGAMENT of the Radius is not, as might be supposed, any distinct ligament, but merely a particular form of that part of the General Capsule.

The

---

* This is the Bursa which I had seen distended with a prodigious quantity of glairy fluid, and producing a tumor upon the shoulder. *Vid.* Book upon the Joints, page 431.

The Coronary Ligament (c) is just that part of the General Capsule, which belongs to the head of the Radius. In attaching itself to the neck of the Radius, it seems a little radiated or pursed up at the root (d); a little higher as at (c), where it goes over the plain button-like head of the Radius, it is braced very firm; it is indeed hard and cartilaginous, particularly hard and smooth within; and at this point, it is especially strengthened by two Accessory Ligaments; the one (m), named the ANTERIOR ACCESSORY LIGAMENT, is hardly to be distinguished from the fore-part of the General Capsule, which is irregular and very lax. This Accessory Ligament is almost mixed with the lower part of the Capsular Ligament; being in fact but a stronger band of the general Capsule, the Capsule being stretched over the point of the Coronoid Process of the Ulna. But there is another strengthening of the Capsule, which forms a more distinct and stronger Accessory Ligament for the Coronary Ligament of the Radius: This Accessory ring of Ligament is marked (n), and rises from the sharp edge of the Coronary Process of the Ulna.

And lastly, the two INTERNAL LATERAL LIGAMENTS, or the strengthenings of the Capsule by slips of Ligament, which come from the Condyle are marked (o o). There are generally two as here represented; but sometimes they are united into one larger Ligament. These two small but strong slips of ligament go from the inner Condyle of the Os Humeri to the root of the Coronoid Process, where it rises from the body of the Ulna.

The INTER-OSSEUS LIGAMENT, which passes betwixt the Radius and Ulna, is marked (p); its stringy fibres are seen, and also the holes by which arteries and veins pass from the fore to the back parts of the fore arm. One particular slip of ligament marked (q), is named CHORDA TRANSVERSALIS CUBITI; and is always found of this form, stretching from the Radius below its Tubercle, to the Coronoid Process of the Ulna.

In the lower part of the same drawing, we have the wrist-joint, where (r) marks the

Scaphoid

Scaphoid Cavity of the Radius (*s*). The moveable Cartilage, small and Triangular, which reprefents the head of the Ulna in this joint (*t*), points out the oval form of this cavity by circumfcribing it; (*u*) fhows the round head of the Os SCAPHOIDES; (*v*) fhows a fimilar round Articulating Surface of the Os LUNARE; and it is here feen, that thefe two are the chief bones on the part of the Carpus, and that they form together an oval head, which, correfponding with the oval form of the Scaphoid Cavity of the Radius (*r*), makes the wrift-joint a regular hinge, not capable of lateral motions.

The Capfule of the wrift which inclofes thefe bones, to form them into a joint, is feen here with its cut edges marked (*t*); for the lines from (*t*) ferve at once to circumfcribe the joint, explaining its oval form, and to mark the cut edges of its Capfule. (*x*) Marks the crofs Ligament of the wrift which binds the tendons down into the deep hollow, which is reprefented here; and (103.) marks the Abductor Pollicis.

PLATE

Pl. I.

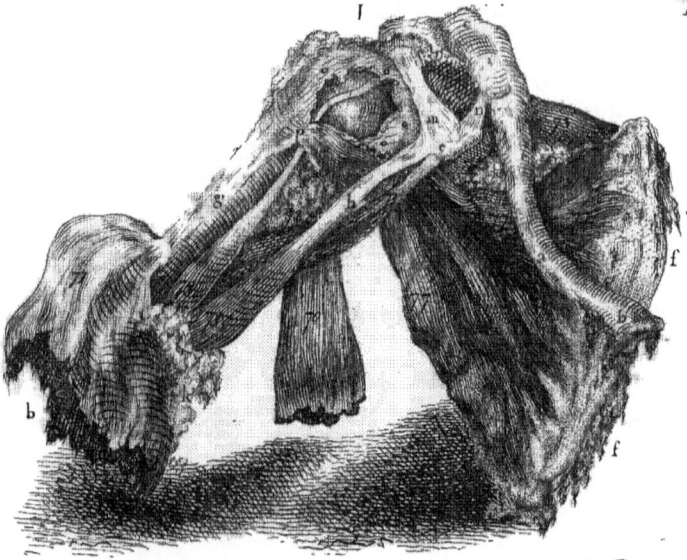

I

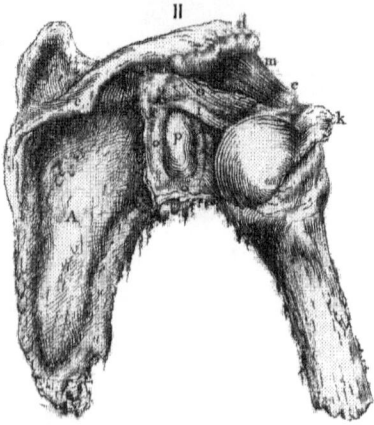

II

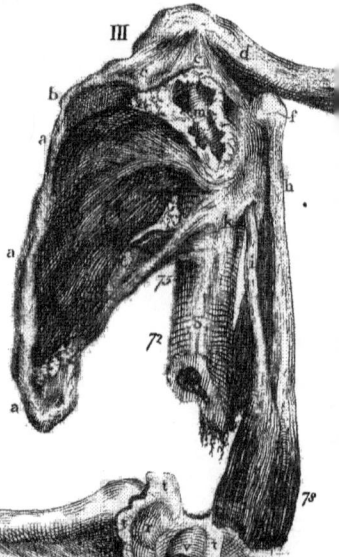

III

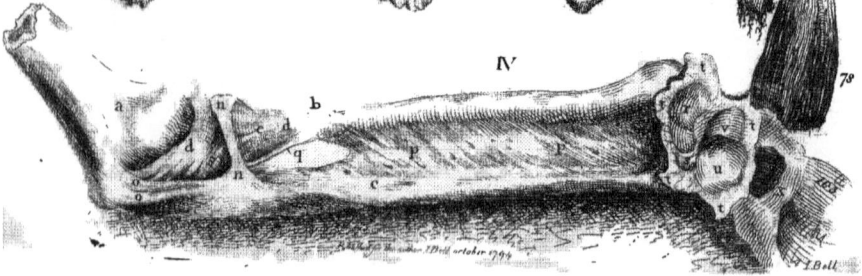

IV

P L A T E II.

This Plate explains the Text Book, from Page 239, to Page 452.

THE two firſt figures of this plate explain the Hip-joint; of which the chief parts are the focket, the head of the bone, the Capfule, and the Central Ligament of the joint.

THE Os ILIUM is marked (*a*); the *creſt* or fpine of the Ilium is marked (*b*); the Poſterior Spinous Proceſſes of the Ilium (*c*); the Anterior Spinous Proceſſes are marked (*d*); the Spinous Procefs of the ISCHIUM, is marked (*e*); and the Tuberoſity of the Ifchium, the loweſt point of the Pelvis, upon which we fit, is marked (*f*); the Ramus or leg of the Ifchium, joining the leg of the Pubis, is marked (*g*); the Thyroid hole (*h*); the Symphiſis Pubis (*i*); and the creſt of the Pubis (*k*); the ſhaft of the thigh bone is marked (*l*); the great Trochanter is marked (*m*); and the head of the bone is marked (7.)

The parts of the joint are marked with numbers, thus,

(1.) Is the bony margin of the Socket where it is formed by the Tuberoſity of the Os Ifchium; there the focket is very deep.

(2.) The Cartilage which encircles the brim of the focket, making it ſtill deeper and more fecure.

(3.) A part of the circle of the focket oppofite to the Thyroid hole, where the focket

2   is

is exceedingly fhallow, or where rather the bony margin of the focket is wanting, and its place is fupplied by a Ligamentous fubftance.

(4.) Is the Capfular Ligament of the hip, which is the ftrongeft in all the body. The thick cut edges of the Burfal Ligament are feen here; and the ligament is feen to come off at (*n*), from the Cartilaginous borders of the Acetabulum, being truely (as it is explained in the defcription of this joint) a continuation of the Perichondrium, or membraneous covering of the Cartilage, confifting of two ~~Cancellæ~~ *Lamella*, one of which comes from the Internal Surface of the Socket, while the other comes from the outer furface of the bone, and both of them are condenfed into the Burfal Ligament.

(5.) Is a ftrengthening of the General Capfule, or what may be called the Acceffory Ligament, coming down from that little Bump which is named the INFERIOR ANTERIOR SPINOUS PROCESS of the Os Ilium; and this Acceffory Ligament is beft feen in figure ii. where the Capfule is preferved entire, chiefly for the purpofe of fhowing this ftrengthening or fupplementary band.

(6.) Is the CENTRAL LIGAMENT, which is commonly called the round ligament, though it is truely of a Triangular form; rifing by a broader bafis at (6.) from the center of the focket, and implanted fmall, neat, and round into that dimple which is feen in the drawings of the thigh bone, in the very center of its globular head; indeed the dimple made by the infertion of this ligament is well feen here at (7.)

(8.) In the deep part of the focket, where this figure is placed, we fee dimples irregularly hollow, which are the beds for lodging the MUCOUS DUCTS of the joint, or what has been called, though not truely, the SYNOVIAL GLAND; and at thefe hollows there are Frenulæ, or little tongues of the inner membrane of the focket, which hold thefe Mucous Dufts in their place; there are alfo little Frenulæ round the neck of the bone, efpecially at its root, which conduft the Mucous Dufts, which lie there.

Thefe are the Frenulæ, or little ligaments, which I meant to enumerate in page 446.

by

by faying " that there are two Internal Ligaments belonging to this joint, *viz.* the " great INTERNAL CENTRAL, or round ligament as it is called, and thefe fmaller " MUCOUS Ligaments."

(9.) Is the root of the Burfal Ligament, for it embraces not merely the head, but alfo the neck of the bone; and it is here explained how the Periofteum (*o*), which is feen torn up from the fhaft of the thigh bone, goes off from the bone at ($\frac{9}{\text{\textit{@}}}$), in the form of Burfal Ligament, fo that the Burfal Ligament and the Periofteum are continuous, being different modifications of one membrane.

F I G U R E S   III. AND IV.

ARE drawings of the outfide of the knee-joint, for explaining the General Capfule of the joint, and efpecially for explaining the ftrengthenings of the Capfule, which are known by the names of Lateral and Pofterior Ligaments.

FIGURE III. fhows the inner fide of the knee-joint, with the great Internal Lateral Ligament. (*a*) Marks the thigh bone; (*b*) the Tibia, and the letter is placed upon that bump, which receives the tendon of all the Extenfor Mufcles; (*c*) the Patella appearing through the tendinous expanfions which cover all the joint.

There is left here a part of the flefhy belly of the Vaftus Internus Mufcle (174.). This belly expands into the form of a thin tendinous fafcia, which goes over the common Capfule of the joint at (*d*), to ftrengthen it. It is at (*e*), that the broad tendon of the Vaftus Internus is inferted into the Patella; and (*f*) is the ftrong LIGAMENT of the PATELLA, which comes down from the pointed lower end of the Patella, which though it is called Ligament, is merely the thick and tough tendon by which all the mufcles, which extend the leg, as the RECTUS, VASTI, and CRURÆUS, are fixed into the knob (*b*), upon the head of the Tibia. (*g*) Marks that margin of the head of the Tibia upon which the Semi-lunar Cartilage plays, and this fharp edge

is

is feen here fhining through the Capfule of the joint. (*i*) Marks the Capfule of the joint itfelf, thin and delicate at this point (by the fide of the Patella). (*k*, Marks the great INTERNAL LATERAL LIGAMENT, which is fometimes named LIGAMENTUM LATUM INTERNUM, from its great breadth. It is not merely a ftrengthening of the common Capfule, as the Lateral Ligaments of the elbow-joint are, but is a firm and diftinct ligament, bright and gliftening with filvery lights upon it like mother of pearl, of full three inches in length, very regular and formal, of a triangular fhape, rifing by a broad bafis from the inner Condyle of the thigh bone, inferted by a fmaller and more pointed end into the head of the Tibia ; and ftretching down the bone, fo as to mix gradually with the Periofteum, and with the General Fafciæ or Tendinous Expanfions, which go out over the fore parts of the Tibia. And that it may be underftood, how little this Ligament is connected with the Capfule, and how fairly it is entitled to the name of Lateral Ligament, I have diffected it fo as to thruft a piece of Bougie (*l*), under the middle of the ligament, where it paffes over the middle of the Capfule. Behind this at (*m*), there is a band of ligament lying, and in the direction of the greater ligament, which might almoft be named as a leffer Internal Lateral Ligament, but which is defcribed only as a ftrengthening of the greater one.

FIGURE IV. at the fame time that it explains the Pofterior Ligaments, reprefents alfo the Lateral Ligaments on the outer fide of the joint. (*a*) Marks the thigh bone ; (*b*) the Tibia ; (*n*) the Fibula ; (*i*) the Burfal Ligament of the joint, fo cut as to expofe the inner Condyle of the thigh bone, naked and fhining.

This Burfal Ligament is ftrengthened every where behind, by irregular ftrings of ligament paffing over it in all directions, but chiefly oblique, and one of thefe oblique Fafciculi or bands is generally fo very ftrong, as to deferve the name of Ligamentum Pofticum. So I have marked the irregular Fafciculi (*o*), and I have marked the more formal Ligament the Ligamentum Pofticum Winflowii (*p*).

The ·

The great LATERAL LIGAMENT on the outer fide of the knee-joint is marked (*q*). It is here feen, that the EXTERNAL LATERAL LIGAMENT is not fo flat as the Internal one, that it does not lie fo fairly as the Internal one upon the fide of the joint, but that it inclines a little towards the back part; and it is feen in the drawing as I have explained it in the book, that the proper External Ligament, the LIGAMENTUM LATERALE EXTERNUM LONGUM (*q*), is a large and ftrong ligament, proceeding from the outer Condyle of the thigh bone, and fixed into the head of the Fibula; but that the LIGAMENTUM EXTERNUM LATERALE BREVIUS vel MINUS (*r*), has not the true form of a Lateral Ligament coming down from the Condyle, but is a mere ftrengthening or outward band of the Capfule, rifing upwards from the knob of the Fibula.

So that in thefe two drawings, iii. and iv. are feen, all the chief parts on the outfide of the knee-joint.

1. The bones as, (*a*) the thigh bone; (*b*) the Tibia; (*c*) the Rotula or Patella; (*n*) the Fibula; and (*f*) the ftrong Ligament of the Patella, a part which is properly arranged with the bones.

2. There is the Capfule and parts connected with it, as (*i*) the thin membrane of the Capfule itfelf; (*d*) the Fafcia or expanding tendon of the Vaftus Internus fpreading over it, to ftrengthen it.

3. The Lateral and Pofterior Ligaments, as (*k*) the INTERNAL LATERAL LIGAMENT, flat, ftrong, and almoft triangular; with a fmall ligament (*m*) to ftrengthen it; (*q*) the great EXTERNAL LATERAL LIGAMENT rounder and more oblique; which (in its turn alfo) is ftrengthened by a fmaller ligament (*r*). And Laftly, the ftrengthenings on the back part of the joint, which are irregular at (*o*), and which form fometimes a more regular Ligament at (*p*), the LIGAMENTUM POSTICUM WINSLOWII.

This Anatomy of the knee-joint is continued in the two firft figures of next plate.

Z   PLATE

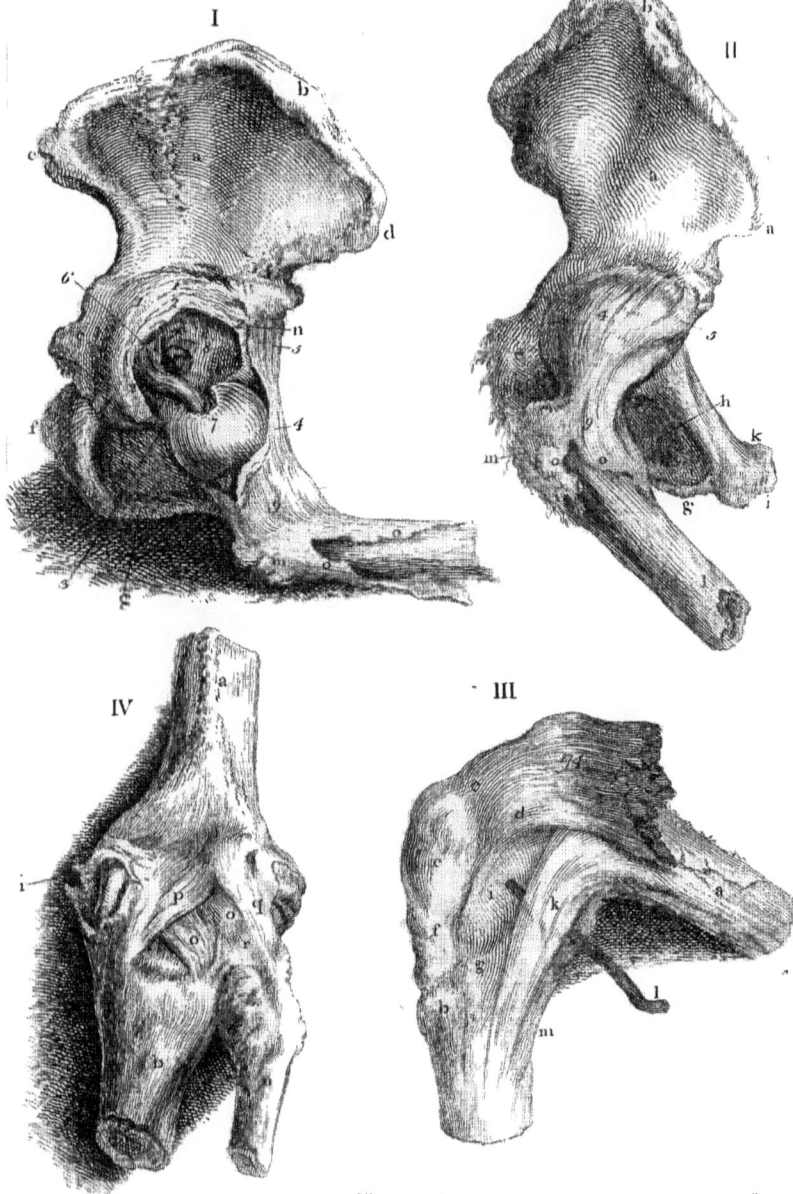

I

II

III

IV

Published ...

P L A T E   III.

This Plate explains the Text Book, from Page 443, to Page 452.

THE Anatomy of the knee-joint is continued in this plate. It explains the internal parts, the knowledge of which is more valuable than of the external parts, in proportion as internal difeafes of this joint are more frequent than luxations, which never happen except in thofe terrible injuries, where all the foft parts belonging to the joint, are entirely torn up by the roots, fo that the limb cannot be faved. The chief parts to be obferved within the joint are the fat, and Mucous Membranes, which lubricate the joint, the Ligaments or Frenulæ, which order and regulate the motions of thefe fatty maffes and fringes., the Semi-lunar Cartilages which, like friction-wheels facilitate the motions of the joint; and Laftly, the great Crucial Ligaments by which the joint is ftrengthened within, the Crucial Ligaments alone being ftronger than the whole of thofe Ligaments which are to be feen on the outfide of the joint.

1. The Fat.

THE fat which is for lubricating the knee-joint, though it is not entirely confined to the circle of the Patella, yet it chiefly furrounds it; and with the fat there are

Z 2   many

many fringes of the Mucous Ducts; much fat is found at each side of the Patella at (*a a*), but the chief collection is at the lower part of the Patella. At (*b*) figure i. this fat appears peeping out from under that ligament, by which its motions are regulated; but at (*b*) in figure ii. the ligament is cut away, and all the fat is freely seen.

This collection of fat and Mucous Ducts makes a rising upon each side of the Patella, marked with a deep, and smooth sulcus round the edge of the bone; and this hanging of the fat on each side of the Patella, is named by WEIDBRIGHT the Ligamentum Alare Majus, where it hangs in the inner side of the Rotula; and Ligamentum Alare Minus, where it projects less at the outside of the Rotula; (*Vid.* (*a a*) figure i.) But all this is quite arbitrary; these are not ligaments, nor do they tie any other part; they are but looser foldings of the inner coat of the Capsule, where it rises over the inner surface of the Patella, and where it holds larger globes of fat, or conducts the fringes of the Mucous Follicules.

2. The Mucous Ligament.

These bundles of fat are tied by a true ligament (*c*), which properly belongs to them. But to understand this ligament and its names, it must be observed, that the two Lunar Cartilages are moveable; that the two horns of the Lunar Cartilages are tacked together by a little Transverse Ligament; and that this Transverse Ligament is again connected with the little mass of fat, which lies under the lower border of the Patella; and lastly, it is to be remembered, that these fatty bundles are chiefly intended for conducting and defending the Mucous Ducts or fringes. Now the ligament (*c*) figure i. which regulates at once the positions of all these parts in the various motions of the joints, has been named " Ligamentum Mucosum," by Vesalius, he referring it to the Mucous Membrane; it is named " the Ligament moving the Semi-lunar Cartilages" by Cheselden; it is named, " Ligamentum Internum

" Longitudinale,"

" Longitudinale" by Walther, becaufe of its running down exactly in the middle
of the joint; it is named not unfrequently " Ligamentum Gracile," from its delicacy. Weidbright feems to call it (in one place at leaft) " Frenulum Pinguedinis
" Glandulofæ;" and he concludes with a queftion, whether this in place of being
a diftinct Ligament be not rather a continuation of his two Aliform Ligaments.

But the nature of this ligament is very diftinct. It is a regular ligament of a very conftant form, and having very curious ufes; it is a ligament tolerably thick, but of a
foft and membranous nature. It is fmall and pointed above as at (d), where it rifes
from the interftice betwixt the two condyles of the thigh bone; it gradually broad-
ens downwards, fo as to acquire rather a triangular form, terminating by a broad
bafe near the root of the patella at (e e). It lies in the fore part, or rather perhaps
in the centre of the joint in the middle behind the patella, and before the Crucial
Ligaments. Its bafis fpreads out into two limbs (e e); one going to the right fide,
and the other to the left, and this forking of it is named by Walther Ligamentum Transversum Semicirculare *; calling the upper and fmaller part of this ligament the Longitudinal Ligament; while he names the bafis and broader part of
the ligament the Tranfverfe Ligament, and it is under this root or tranfverfe part
of the mucous ligament that the fat which it confines is feen peeping out at (b).

This ligament then, (which in place of dividing thus curioufly into Longitudinal and
Tranfverfe or Alar ligaments, may be defcribed under the general title of Mucous
Ligament), is of confiderable fize, being almoft of the thicknefs of the little finger, and
is the part that is feen when the joint is firft opened; not firm and hard like thofe
ligaments which tie the bones, but foft, delicate, and membranous, fit for its office of
conducting the mucous ducts in fafety, and regulating the motions of the fatty bundles. It is fmall at (d), where it comes off from the great Sulcus betwixt the condyles.

* So Walther names as Tranfverfe Ligament thofe parts which Weidbright marks by the names of
Ligamentum Alare Majus and Minus.

dyles. It grows broad at its root, being there so large as to fill up all the empty
space in the joint. It assumes at its lower part a triangular or prismatic form, with
one flat side directly forwards, and the other angle of the prism looking backwards in
the joint, and covering the crucial ligaments which lie in the back part of the cavity. After enlarging at its basis, it degenerates into a soft mucous or membranous covering for the fat and mucous glands; thus it is connected at its root
with the lower edge of the patella; with the fat and mucous fringes, and with the
fore horns of the Semilunar Cartilages. So that this ligament moves in every motion of the joint, as the thigh-bone from which it rises moves, it is moved the more
from its connection with the patella, and as this ligament moves along with the
patella, it in its turn moves the Semilunar Cartilages and the bundles of fat, and
keeps them fixed, or draws them forwards; for were the fat permitted to move backwards, it would be bruised directly betwixt the bones with a force that would destroy
it; and thus the mucous ducts not only by the elasticity of the fat which surrounds
them, start out from betwixt the bones when they press too closely; but the fat together with all the glands which belong to it is so held forward by this mucous ligament as to lie always in the free and open part of the joint.

This ligament was thought by the ancients to be sometimes wanting, though this
cannot be true of a part so essential to the sound constitution and free motions of
the joint. It is believed by some, that it may be torn in sudden and violent
bendings of the knee; it surely is the part the most subject to disease, since we find it
in ulcerated joints quite coroded. It is plain that this part must be most peculiarly
subject to inflame, since it is continually working in every motion of the joint; it is
not only delicate in itself, but is connected with all the more delicate parts; for the inner membrane of the capsule is continuous with this Mucous Ligament; the fat that
surrounds the patella is continuous with it; it conducts the fringes or ducts of the chief
mucous glands; it is itself a secreting surface, and the moveable or Semilunar Carti-

lages

lages are tied to it; by all which circumſtances it becomes too important in the œ. conomy and diſeaſes of this delicate joint to be paſſed ſlightly over.

3. THE MOVEABLE CARTILAGES.

The two MOVEABLE CARTILAGES are not ſeen in Fig. i. becauſe the mucous ligament which covers them is entire. In Fig. ii. they are marked (m m). The letters (m m) touch the outer edges of the cartilages, where their outer margins adhere to the inner ſurface of the capſule.

The parts and connexions of theſe cartilages are better explained in Fig. iii. where (m m) ſtill mark the outer circles which adhere to the inner ſurface of the capſule. The letters (n n) mark the thinner edges, and ſhow the ſpace in the center of each cartilage which holds the condyle of the thigh-bone. (p p) Mark the two poſterior horns and the little tags of ligament by which they are tied to the crucial ligaments behind. And (q q) mark the two anterior horns, and the little tags of ligament by which they are tied to the root of the mucous ligament before. And (r) marks a little croſs ligament by which the two anterior horns are connected with each other, and which is named LIGAMENTUM TRANSVERSALE COMMUNE.

4. THE CRUCIAL LIGAMENTS

Are well ſeen in Fig. ii. where (c) marks the part from which the pointed origin of the mucous ligament was cut away. And by cutting away that ligament, the Crucial Ligaments which, in Fig. i. are covered by the mucous or central ligaments, are in this drawing brought into view

The Crucial Ligaments lie both in the back part of the joint, and touch that part of the Capſule, which lies in the Ham; but one of them (s) lies behind, whence it is called the Poſterior Ligament, and the other (t) though it lies flat upon the Poſterior

Ligament,

Ligament, and in contact with it; yet being before it, is named the Anterior Ligament.

The reason of this Anterior Ligament being represented as coming so far forwards as to touch in a manner the root of the Patella, is plainly this; that to take a sure hold of the Tibia it does actually rise over the tubercle in the center of the joint, and goes out flat over all the face of the joint, and the reason of the Posterior Ligament seeming to follow this one, and to come also far forwards in the joint, is, that the ligaments of the horns of the Lunar Cartilages climb upon the fore-part of the Posterior Ligament, and so it is more properly the Ligament of the Lunar Cartilage that is seen at (*u*), while the head only of the Posterior Crucial Ligament is seen at (*s*).—— But both the true direction and extent of these ligaments and their true office will be better understood by the following plan; for there is this one thing very singular in the effect of these ligaments, that it is not the Posterior Ligament that checks the leg and prevents it going too far forwards; nor the Anterior Ligament that prevents it being strained backwards, but quite the reverse; for the Posterior Ligament is most stretched when the knee is bended; the Anterior Ligament again is stretched when the leg is extended.

FIGURE I. Shows the leg extended.
FIGURE II. Shows the knee bent.

In Figure 1st, (*a*) is the Thigh-bone; (*b*) the Inner Condyle; (*c*) the Outer Condyle; (*d*) the head of the Tibia; (*e*) the knob in the center of the Knee-joint; and (1) is the Anterior Ligament arising from the Outer Condyle, (viz. the one nearest the eye in this drawing), and going out over the fore-part of the Tibia, and inserted properly into that hollow (*f*), which receives the Condyle; (2) is the Posterior Ligament, rising rather from the center of the Thigh-bone betwixt the Condyles, and going down over the back-part of the Tibia at (*g*).

2   And

And in figure ii. it is plain by the change of the pofition of the bones, that when the knee is bent, the Pofterior Ligament (2.) is ftretched, and the Anterior (1.) re-laxed. And of courfe, as in figure i. that when the leg is extended, the Anterior Ligament (1.) will be ftretched, and the Pofterior (2.) relaxed.

A a

In

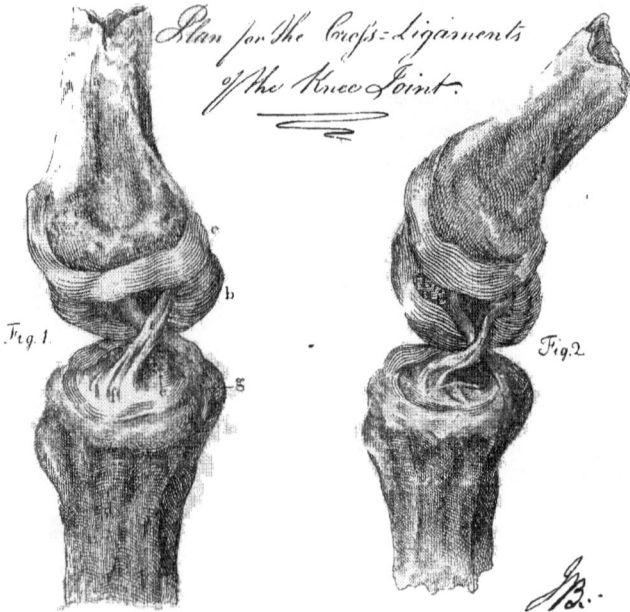

Plan for the Crofs-Ligaments of the Knee Joint.

Fig. 1.

Fig. 2.

In thefe three drawings, all the internal parts of the knee-joint are explained.

1. The FAT which is collected chiefly round the Patella, which perhaps does not exude nor mix with the fluid of the joint, but ferves rather by its Lubricity and Elaftic nature, to conduct and defend the fringes or Mucous Ducts.

2. The MUCOUS LIGAMENT, which is the firft part that is feen upon opening the joint; which lies in the center of the joint; is of a foft and mucous nature; conducts many of the Mucous Fringes; and which, defcending from the middle of the thigh bone betwixt the Condyles, is attached to the lower edge of the Patella, and to the Semi-lunar Ligaments, and fo it moves along with the Patella, and moves in its turn the Cartilages and the fat. It regulates the motions of the Cartilages, and it draws forwards the fat, preventing it going backwards, fo as to be bruifed betwixt the bones.

3. The SEMI-LUNAR CARTILAGES, which are like the labels which are put round the neck of a wine flafk. They are tied at the horns by ligaments, as the label is hung by its chain; lie flat upon the Tibia, to facilitate its motions, and enable, at the fame time, the Condyles of the thigh bone to change their centers of motion, according to the various poftures of the joint.

4. The CROSS LIGAMENTS, which are very thick, and ftrong, lie chiefly in the back part of the joint, and by their going the one over the face of the Tibia, and the other down along the back of the bone, they limit both its motions, the one checking it in too violent bendings of the knee, the other limiting its extenfions. So that the motions forwards and backwards are limited by thefe Crofs Ligaments within the joint, while it is fecured from irregular Lateral motions by the ftrong Lateral Ligaments without.

FIGURES

F I G U R E S   IV.   AND   V.

EXPLAIN the Ligaments of the ancle joint, and of the foot. All the great Ligaments belonging to the ancle joint, or to the Tarfal Bones are drawn in figure iv. and in figure V. are feen the two great ligaments lying in the fole of the foot.

F I G U R E   IV.

THE Ligaments belonging to the ancle joint are thefe,

(1.) A ftrong Ligament tying the Fibula to the Tibia. It is large and very ftrong; commonly it is divided, as here, into two, fometimes into three flips; fometimes they all adhere. It is named the LIGAMENTUM ANTICUM SUPERIUS. There is on the back part of the Fibula a ligamentous membrane, which is like this one, and is named Ligamentum Fibulae Pofticum Superius.

Thefe ligaments connect the Tibia and Fibula fo firmly to each other, that they are as one bone with two proceffes, viz. the inner and outer ancles.

(2.) Is the MIDDLE PERPENDICULAR LIGAMENT, a very ftrong ligament, which defcends directly from the point of the outer ancle, to tie it firmly to the fide of the Os Calcis. There are three ligaments tying the outer ancle to the foot; viz. firft, this middle one; fecond, the anterior one; and, third, one behind the joint, a pofterior ligament, which is not feen. This Middle Perpendicular Ligament, fo named from its pofition, defcends directly from the very point of the outer ancle, and it is implanted into the fide of the heel bone. It holds the ancle from yielding to one fide, and from bending too much; affifting rather the pofterior ligament than the anterior one. It lies clofe upon the Capfule, and ftrengthens it; while the tendons of the Peronaei Mufcles glide and rub acrofs it.

A a 2

(3.) The

(3.) The ANTERIOR LIGAMENT of the outer ancle is for tying the outer ancle to the Aftragalus, as the perpendicular one ties it to the heel bone. It goes fometimes in two diftinct bands, as reprefented here. Very often they are fcarcely divided; it appearing as one ftrong uniform ligament, white and gliftening, paffing obliquely forwards from the loweft point of the Fibula to the neck of the Aftragalus.

Thefe three are the chief ligaments of the ancle; and the order of ligaments which come next, is of thofe which tie the Aftragalus to the Os Calcis and to the Os Naviculare.

1ft, (a) Is a ligament, or rather two or three ligaments, which crofs the great hole, which, in the drawings of the bones of the Tarfus, is marked with a pencil thruft up through it. This is called the Cavitas Sinuofa; and fo thefe irregular ligaments are named Ligamenta, or APARATUS LIGAMENTOSUS CAVITATIS SINUOSÆ. They are merely irregular ligaments, lying deep in this hollow, and tying the Aftragalus to the Os Calcis.

2d, (b) Is a ligament which ties the Aftragalus to the Os Naviculare. It begins at the neck of the Aftragalus; touches the Os Naviculare; goes ftill forwards, and fpreads a little upon the cuneiform bones; and, from this expanding form, is named LIGAMENTUM LATUM. Though there are feveral bands of ligament on the inner fide, they are not fo particular, nor fo formal in their fhapes or ufes, as to have any appropriated name.

3d, (c) There are ligaments tying the Os Calcis, in its turn, to the Os Naviculare and to the Os Cuboides. The letter (c) is placed upon that prominent point of the Os Calcis whence thofe ligaments go off; and they go fomewhat in a ftar-like form, juft as I have drawn them, and not very diftinct. And thofe bands which go upwards tie the Os Calcis to the Os Naviculare;—thofe which go downwards tie it to the Os Cuboides; for the chief articulation of the heel-bone is with the Os Cuboides.

4th, (d) There goes a little flip of ligament, not much noticed from this fame point of

the

the heel-bone, to that part (*e*) of the metatarfal bone of the little toe, which is very fharp and prominent; and is in all pofitions and drawings the moft remarkable point in the foot.

The ligaments again, which tie the feveral bones of the Tarfus, as the cuboid and cuneiform bones, together, are flat, fhining, ftar-like, and very numerous; and, from their lying upon the back of the foot, are named LIGAMENTA PLANA DORSALIA. They are marked (*rrr*); and are too irregular in their form, and too general in their ufes, to need any more accurate indication; for thefe are the ligaments which are fo croffed and interwoven, " that they form what we may call a web of liga-" ments, confifting of fhining and ftar-like bundles," of a cartilaginous hardnefs, adhering clofely to the whole furface, and paffing from bone to bone over all the furface of the foot. (*t*) Is the Ligamentum Longum, which is marked 3. in the 5th drawing, and is explained in the letter prefs of that figure.

The ligaments which tie together the Tarfus and Metatarfus are alfo feen here, at the roots of the metatarfal bones. There are lateral ligaments which tie each metatarfal bone to the one next it. But the ligaments which appear chiefly upon this upper furface, are a continuation of the irregular web of ligament belonging to the Tarfal bones; and as this web takes particular fhapes in paffing along to the feveral heads of the Metatarfal bones, thefe are beft named, in general terms, LIGAMENTA DORSALIA, the Dorfal Ligaments of the Metatarfal bones; and they are marked (*sss*).

In FIGURE V.

THE Ancle joint is feen opened. The Tibia and Fibula (*a* & *b*) are turned backwards. Their ftrong ligament (*c*), which binds them together, is feen; the Capfule, which is clean diffected, is marked (*d*), which fhows its cut edges. (*e*) Shows

that

that it is a reflection of the Capsule that lines the cavity of the joint; and the process (*f*) of the *inner* ancle being turned back, the great head, or the cartilaginous pulley of the Aftragalus (*g*), is expofed covered with its fmooth cartilage. The flat fide of the Aftragalus within the joint is alfo feen at (*b*), where it was embraced by the inner ancle or procefs of the Tibia (*f*). There is but one ligament to be noticed in this drawing; for

1ft, Is a band very ftrong indeed, which paffes from the Aftragalus to the Os Calcis. It has, as is feen here, the diftinct form of a ligament. It ties the Aftragalus and Os Calcis ftrongly together; and fo it has alfo the office as well as the mere form of a ligament. But it often happens, that the tendon of the Flexor Pollicis runs through this ring; therefore its office as a ligament (which it truly is) is very little noticed.

2d, There is a ligament of the inner ancle, like the perpendicular ligament of the outer ancle. It is of a triangular form; and is hence named Ligamentum Deltoides. A procefs of this ligament binds down the Tendons of the Tibialis Pofticus, and of the common flexor of the toes. Therefore the ligament marked (2), at the fame time that it binds the bones of the foot together, holds down the flexor tendons.

3d, The figure (3) marks the great ligament of the fole of the foot. It proceeds fmaller from the point of the heel bone; it enlarges towards its infertion into the Os Cuboides. It binds thefe two bones particularly; and, by binding them, it fupports very powerfully the whole arch of the foot; and this ligament, which is alfo very thick and ftrong, is of fuch particular length, (the longeft ligament of all the Tarfus), that it is called Ligamentum Calcis Longius. It is feen under the edge of the foot in the drawing, figure iv. marked (*t*).

But the trueft fupport of any joint is not its ligaments fo much as the mufcles which bend it; and it is thus with all the flexor mufcles which pafs under this great arch of the foot—How could the arch of the foot be fuftained, by ligaments of any kind, under

2   the

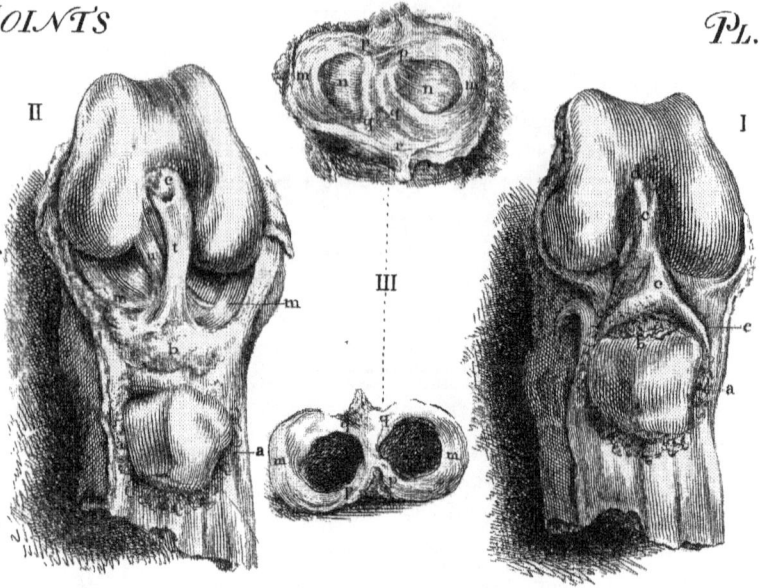

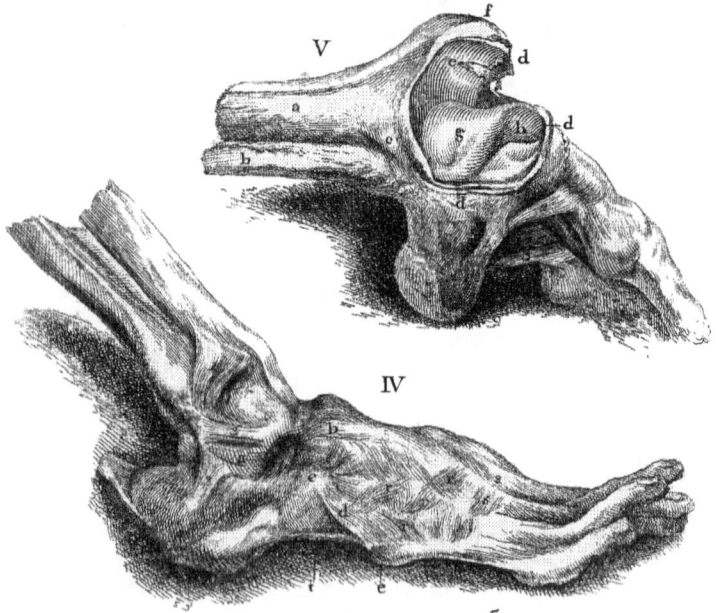

Pl. III.

II

III

I

V

IV

Published as the act directs 1.st October 1794

the whole weight of the body, and its exertions? Surely it could not be fuftained
otherwife than by the ftrong action of the Tibialis Pofticus and the flexor mufcles of
the toes; and when a man ftands under a burden, as well as when he walks, this
arch is fuftained by the continual action of thofe mufcles the tendons of which pafs
under the arch.

F I N I S.

www.ingramcontent.com/pod-product-compliance
Lightning Source LLC
Chambersburg PA
CBHW021947220326

41599CB00012BA/1232